Fertility and Obstetrics in Cattle

LIBRARY OF VETERINARY PRACTICE

EDITORS

J.B. SUTTON JP, MRCVS

S.T. SWIFT MA, VetMB, CertSAC

LIBRARY OF VETERINARY PRACTICE

Fertility and Obstetrics in Cattle

Second Edition

D.E. NOAKES
BVetMed, PhD, FRCVS, DVReprod
Department of Farm Animal and Equine Medicine and Surgery
The Royal Veterinary College
University of London

Blackwell
Science

© 1986, 1997 by
Blackwell Science Ltd
Editorial Offices:
Osney Mead, Oxford OX2 0EL
25 John Street, London WC1N 2BL
23 Ainslie Place, Edinburgh EH3 6AJ
238 Main Street, Cambridge
  Massachusetts 02142, USA
54 University Street, Carlton
  Victoria 3053, Australia

Other Editorial Offices:
Arnette Blackwell SA
  224, Boulevard Saint Germain
  75007 Paris, France

Blackwell Wissenschafts-Verlag GmbH
  Kurfürstendamm 57
  10707 Berlin, Germany

  Zehetnergasse 6
  A-1140 Wien
  Austria

First edition published 1986
Second edition published 1997

Set in 10 on 12 pt Souvenir
by DP Photosetting, Aylesbury, Bucks
Printed and bound in Great Britain by
The University Press, Cambridge.

The Blackwell Science logo is a trade mark of
Blackwell Science Ltd, registered at the
United Kingdom Trade Marks Registry

DISTRIBUTORS

Marston Book Services Ltd
PO Box 269
Abingdon
Oxon OX14 4YN
(*Orders:* Tel: 01235 465500
         Fax: 01235 465555)

USA
Blackwell Science, Inc.
238 Main Street
Cambridge, MA 02142
(*Orders:* Tel: 800 215-1000
              617 876-7000
         Fax: 617 492-5263)

Canada
Copp Clark, Ltd
2775 Matheson Blvd East
Mississauga, Ontario
Canada, L4W 4P7
(*Orders:* Tel: 800 263-4374
              905 238-6074)

Australia
Blackwell Science Pty Ltd
54 University Street
Carlton, Victoria 3053
(*Orders:* Tel: 03 9347 0300
         Fax: 03 9347 5001)

A catalogue record for this title is available
from the British Library

ISBN 0-632-04083-1

Library of Congress
Cataloging-in-Publication Data
Noakes, David E.
    Fertility and obstetrics in cattle/D.E.
Noakes.—2nd ed.
    p. cm.—(Library of veterinary
practice)
    Includes bibliographical references
(p.   ) and index.
    ISBN 0-632-04083-1 (pbk.)
    1. Cattle—Fertility.   2. Cattle—
Reproduction.   3. Veterinary obstetrics.
4. Veterinary gynecology.   I. Title.
II. Series.
SF768.2.C3N63   1997
636.2′0898—dc20   96-43821
                                CIP

Contents

Preface   *xiii*
List of Abbreviations   *xiv*

Part 1:   The Female   **1**

1   Normal Non-pregnant Animal   **3**

    1.1   Puberty   3
    1.2   Factors influencing the time of onset of puberty   3
    1.3   Cyclical ovarian activity   4
    1.4   Stages of the oestrous cycle   4
    1.5   Ovarian changes during the cycle   4
    1.6   Hormones produced by the ovary   5
    1.7   Hormonal changes during the oestrous cycle   6
    1.8   Oestrus and its detection   8
        Signs of oestrus   8
        Methods of detection   9
    1.9   Aids to improving oestrus detection   9
    1.10   Methods of artificially controlling the oestrous cycle   11
    1.11   Shortening the lifespan of the corpus luteum   11
    1.12   Progestagens – principles of use   11
        Synchronisation with a progesterone-releasing
        intravaginal device (PRID)   12
        Synchronisation with an intravaginal
        progesterone-releasing device (CIDR)   13
        Synchronisation with Norgestamet   13
    1.13   Synchronisation of oestrus with $PGF_2\alpha$ or analogues   14
        Reasons for poor synchronisation   14
        Reasons for poor conception rates (pregnancy rates)   15
        A compromise regimen   15
        Prostaglandins and analogues available for cattle   15
    1.14   Clinical examination of the genital system   15
        External clinical examination   15
        Vaginal examination using a speculum   16

	Manual examination of the vagina	17
	Rectal palpation	17
1.15	Ultrasonography	23
	Principle	23
	Technique	24
	Identification of structures	27

2 Normal Pregnancy — **28**

2.1	Ovulation	28
2.2	Fertilisation	28
2.3	Embryonic development	29
2.4	Fetal membranes	29
2.5	Fetal fluids	31
2.6	Fetal growth and crown–rump lengths	31
2.7	Estimation of fetal age	32
2.8	Placenta	32
2.9	Maternal recognition of pregnancy	33
2.10	Endocrinology of pregnancy	33
2.11	Methods of pregnancy diagnosis	33
2.12	Accuracy of pregnancy diagnosis by rectal palpation	36

3 Normal Parturition — **37**

3.1	Duration of pregnancy	37
3.2	Birth weight	37
3.3	Fetal growth rate	38
3.4	Twinning and multiples	38
3.5	Freemartins	38
	Diagnosis of freemartins	38
3.6	Initiation of parturition	39
3.7	Signs of impending calving	39
3.8	First stage of parturition	40
3.9	Second stage of parturition	40
3.10	Third stage of parturition	40
3.11	Calving environment	41
3.12	Premature induction of calving	41
	Hormones used in induction	41
	Indications for induction	42
	Requirements	42
	Procedures	42
	Problems	42
3.13	Delaying calving	43

4 Care of the New-born Calf — **44**

| 4.1 | Introduction | 44 |
| 4.2 | Adaptation to the environment | 44 |

4.3	Procedures following the birth of the calf	44
4.4	Problems following birth	45
4.5	Weakly calves	45

5 The Post-partum Period (Puerperium) **46**

5.1	Introduction	46
5.2	Return of normal cyclical ovarian activity	46
5.3	Methods of determining return of cyclical activity	47
5.4	Factors influencing return of cyclical activity	47
5.5	Involution	47
	Factors influencing rate of involution	48
5.6	Regeneration of the endometrium	48
	Factors delaying regeneration of the endometrium	49
5.7	Bacterial contamination	49
5.8	Elimination of bacterial contamination	49
	Factors interfering with the elimination of bacteria	50
5.9	Fertility postpartum	50

6 Lactation **51**

6.1	Normal mammary development	51
6.2	Lactogenesis	51
6.3	Milk let-down	52
	Induction of let-down	52
6.4	Artificial induction of lactation	52
	Method A	52
	Method B	53
	Results	53
	Indications	53

7 Fertility and Infertility in the Cow **54**

7.1	Definitions	54
7.2	Infertility and culling	54
7.3	Expectations for fertility – the individual cow	54
7.4	The reasons for a 12-month interval between calvings	55
7.5	Factors responsible for infertility	55
7.6	No signs of oestrus – approach and clinical examination	55
	Heifers	56
	Heifers and cows	56
7.7	Regular return to oestrus	59
	Failure of fertilisation	60
	Early embryonic death	63
7.8	Short interoestrous interval	64
7.9	Prolonged interoestrous interval	65

7.10	Evaluating herd fertility	65
7.11	Monitoring and maintaining good fertility	69
	Accurate and permanent records	69
	Cows requiring examination	69
	Frequency of veterinary visits	70
	Recording systems	70

8   Problems During Pregnancy   **71**

8.1	Prenatal death	71
	Early embryonic death	71
	Late embryonic death	71
8.2	Causes of embryonic death	71
	Specific infectious agents responsible for embryonic death	72
8.3	Fetal death	72
8.4	Fetal mummification	72
8.5	Abortion	73
	Frequency	73
8.6	Action to be taken following an abortion	74
	Abortions and herd records	74
8.7	Causes of abortion	74
	Infectious causes of abortion	74
	Non-infectious causes of abortion	77
8.8	Diagnosis of causes of abortion	77
8.9	Stillbirth	78
8.10	Fetal maceration	78
8.11	Congenital abnormalities	79
	Causes	79
	Some common congenital abnormalities and their causes	79
8.12	Cervico-vaginal prolapse	82
	Causes	82
	Diagnosis and prognosis	83
	Treatment	83
8.13	Uterine torsion	83
8.14	Uterine rupture	84
8.15	Hydrops amnii and hydrops allantois	85

9   Dystocia   **86**

9.1	Definition	86
9.2	Incidence	86
9.3	Causes	86
9.4	Dealing with a case of dystocia	86
9.5	Clinical examination	87
9.6	Diagnosis	87

9.7	Treatment	88
	Correction of faulty disposition	88
	Traction	89
	Fetotomy (embryotomy)	89
	Caesarean operation	91
9.8	Specific causes of dystocia – Group 1	91
	Feto-maternal disproportion	91
	Partial (or incomplete) cervical dilatation	92
	Vulval or vaginal stricture	93
	Soft tissue obstructions	93
	Bony defects of the pelvis	93
	Uterine torsion	93
	Simultaneous presentation of twins	94
	Monsters (congenitally deformed calves)	94
	Abnormal disposition	95
	Abnormal disposition due to postural abnormalities	95
	Abnormal disposition due to positional abnormalities	96
	Abnormal disposition due to presentational abnormalities	96
9.9	Specific causes of dystocia – Group 2	97
	Uterine rupture	97
	Uterine torsion	97
	Incomplete cervical dilatation	97
	Uterine inertia	97
	Ventral deviation or displacement of the uterus	98
10	**Placental Retention**	**99**
10.1	Introduction	99
10.2	Incidence	99
10.3	Causes	99
10.4	Consequences	100
10.5	Treatment	100
11	**Problems During the Puerperium**	**102**
11.1	Introduction	102
11.2	Lacerations of the vulva and vagina	102
	Vaginal lacerations	102
	Vulval lacerations	102
11.3	Contusions of the genital tract	104
11.4	Haematomas	104
11.5	Peripheral nerve damage	104
11.6	Uterine tears	104
11.7	Uterine prolapse	105
11.8	Acute metritis	107

| | 11.9 | Chronic endometritis | 107 |
| | 11.10 | Pyometra | 108 |

12		**Manipulation of Reproduction**	**110**
	12.1	Twinning and multiple ovulations	110
		Desirability of inducing twinning	110
	12.2	Embryo transfer	110
		Applications of embryo transfer	110
		Requirements for successful embryo transfer	111
		Conduct of embryo transfer	111
		Selection of the donor	111
		Selection of recipients	111
		Superovulatory hormones	112
		Preparation and superovulation of the donor	112
		Preparation of recipients	113
		Collection of embryos	113
		Recovery of the embryos	116
		Transfer of the embryos	116
	12.3	Freezing and storage of embryos	117
	12.4	Micromanipulation of embryos	117
	12.5	*In vitro* maturation and fertilisation of oocytes	117

| **Part 2:** | | **The Male** | **119** |

13		**Normal Male Animal**	**121**
	13.1	Reproductive anatomy of the bull	121
		The testes – structure and function	121
		Endocrine function	121
		Epididymis	122
		Ductus deferens and ampulla	123
		Prostate gland	123
		Vesicular glands (seminal vesicles)	123
		Bulbo-urethral glands	124
		The penis	124
	13.2	Puberty	124
	13.3	Copulatory behaviour	125
	13.4	Clinical examination of the bull for breeding fitness	125
	13.5	Methods of semen collection	126
	13.6	Semen composition	127
	13.7	Semen evaluation	128
	13.8	Frequency of natural service	128

14   Artificial Insemination   **129**

   14.1   Introduction   129
          Advantages   129
          Disadvantages   129
   14.2   Semen collection   130
   14.3   Handling and processing of semen –
          general principles   130
          Processing procedure   130
          Thawing before insemination   131
   14.4   Insemination technique   131
          Timing of insemination   132
   14.5   Selection and care of bulls at AI centres   133
   14.6   Regulations concerning the use of AI in the UK   133
   14.7   Methods of assessing the efficiency of AI   134
   14.8   Poor results from AI   134

15   Infertility in the Bull   **135**

   15.1   General considerations   135
   15.2   Method of investigation   135
   15.3   Loss or lack of libido   135
          Treatment of poor libido   136
   15.4   Impotence   136
   15.5   Impotence associated with failure to protrude
          the penis   136
   15.6   Impotence associated with failure of intromission   137
   15.7   Impotence associated with non-ejaculation   138
   15.8   Reduction in, or failure of, fertilisation   138

Further reading   *140*

Index   *141*

Preface

The first edition of this book was intended primarily as an immediate source of reference and information for veterinary students, veterinary surgeons and anyone working with cattle. Judging by the response of the reviewers, together with comments from my own students and colleagues, this object seems to have been fulfilled. The second edition still aims to satisfy these criteria; it is not intended to be a detailed treatise on the subject and, in the interests of brevity, a certain dogmatism will prevail. Since the publication of the first edition, there have been a number of major developments in cattle reproduction, not least the widespread use of diagnostic B-mode ultrasonography. In addition, there has been a vast amount of new work published in scientific and clinical journals. There is an ever-increasing quantity of high quality literature on cattle reproduction and readers are urged to look elsewhere for other opinions and philosophies; a revised list of further reading will be found at the end of the book.

My initial interest in the subject was stimulated as a boy by the many days spent helping my late uncle with his herd of dairy Shorthorns, and maintained by the teaching of Emeritus Professor Geoffrey Arthur at the Royal Veterinary College; the same interest and enthusiasm still prevails. I must thank the authors of the many books and papers that I have read, my friends and colleagues in the veterinary profession, and the reviewers of the first edition for their helpful comments, particularly Roger Blowey.

Finally, I wish to thank Rosemary Forster for secretarial assistance, the library staff at the Royal Veterinary College for their helpful cooperation, and Richard Miles, Janet Prescott and Julie Musk at Blackwell Science, for their patience and my wife for her hours of isolation whilst I revised the book.

David Noakes

List of Abbreviations

ABP	androgen binding protein
ACTH	adrenocorticotrophic hormone
ADH	antidiuretic hormone
AI	artificial insemination
AV	artificial vagina
bFSH	bovine follicular stimulating hormone
BVD	bovine viral diarrhoea
BVD-1	bovine herpes virus 1
CCP	corpora cavernosa penis
CL	corpus luteum
CRL	crown–rump length
CSP	corpus spongiosum penis
eCG	equine chorionic gonadotrophin
EPS	enriched phosphate-buffered saline
FSH	follicular stimulating hormone
GnRH	gonadotrophin releasing hormone
hCG	human chorionic gonadotrophin
hMG	human monopausal gonadotrophin
IBR	infectious bovine rhinotracheitis
LH	luteinising hormone
LHRH	luteinising hormone releasing hormone
PSPB	pregnancy-specific protein B

Part 1
The Female

1 Normal Non-pregnant Animal

1.1 PUBERTY

At birth, the ovaries of the heifer contain up to 150 000 primordial follicles. During the prepubertal period there are waves of follicular growth and regression, as occurs in postpubertal animals; however, although the maximum size of dominant follicles can be as great as 12 mm in diameter, they all become atretic.

The onset of puberty is identified by the occurrence of regular cyclical ovarian activity. The hypothalamus, in particular the preoptic and the medial basal areas, has a primary role in controlling the transition to sexual maturity. The neurones in the preoptic area, as they mature, become less sensitive to the inhibitory effect of the low levels of oestradiol secreted by the follicles. As a result, gonadotrophin releasing hormone (GnRH – see section 1.7) is produced which stimulates the secretion of luteinising hormone (LH) which induces follicular maturation, ovulation and thus the onset of cyclical ovarian activity. Changes in follicular stimulating hormone (FSH) appear not to be involved in the onset of puberty.

Puberty occurs between 7 and 18 months of age when dairy heifers have reached 35% and beef heifers 40% of mature body weight. In rare instances, heifers have been reported as reaching puberty as early as 3 months.

1.2 FACTORS INFLUENCING THE TIME OF ONSET OF PUBERTY

- Genotype; relationship between age at puberty and subsequent milk yield as an adult within certain breeds.
- Season of year; earlier in Brahman heifers in spring and summer.
- Growth; slower growth delays onset of puberty.
- Nutrition; feeding high energy levels can advance the age of puberty.
- Social cues; bull presence can advance the age of puberty.
- Climate; delayed onset in Mediterranean and tropical compared with temperate climates.
- Disease; can delay the onset, particularly if growth rate is affected.

1.3 CYCLICAL OVARIAN ACTIVITY

The cow is polyoestrous with recurring cycles on average every 21 days (range 18–24); the interval between is referred to as the interoestrous interval. Cyclical activity is absent before the onset of puberty, during pregnancy and for a short period after calving (see section 5.1).

1.4 STAGES OF THE OESTROUS CYCLE

The only clearly definable stage is that of *oestrus* when the cow or heifer will stand to be served by the bull; this lasts on average 15 h (range 2–30 h). Ovulation occurs about 15 h after the end of oestrus.

The rest of the cycle may be divided into *pro-oestrus, meteostrus and dioestrus*, but these are not clearly defined.

- Pro-oestrus is the stage before oestrus when there is increased follicular growth and regression of the corpus luteum (CL), and the genital system is ceasing to be under the domination of the hormone progesterone. There are some behavioural signs that indicate the approach of oestrus, such as increased frequency of attempts to mount other cows.
- Metoestrus is the period after the end of oestrus when the follicle matures, ovulates and the CL starts to develop.
- Dioestrus is the stage when the CL is the dominant structure. Its effect is exerted by the hormone progesterone.

1.5 OVARIAN CHANGES DURING THE CYCLE

With the onset of puberty waves of follicular growth and development occur throughout the entire oestrous cycle culminating in ovulation and the release of the oocyte.

Several different categories of follicles are present on the ovaries:

- Primordial follicles, which are non-growing, 100 μm in diameter.
- Primary follicles, which are early growing follicles in which the oocyte is surrounded by a single layer of cuboidal granulosa cells.
- Secondary follicles, in which the oocyte is surrounded by many layers of cells, including thecal cells.
- Tertiary or antral follicles, in which the antral cavity has developed within the many layers of cells. This occurs when they are 0.4–0.8 mm in diameter.

Follicular growth and development (folliculogenesis) is dependent upon gonadotrophin as well as intra-ovarian and intrafollicular mechanisms; from the formation of an antral follicle to reaching a preovulatory size takes about 40 days.

The waves of follicular growth are induced by surges of the gonado-trophin hormone FSH which occur before the development of 4–5 mm follicles. In some individuals there are two, and in others three, FSH surges which stimulate either two or three waves of follicular growth, respectively. Cows or heifers with three waves will have longer (normal) interoestrous intervals than cows with two. Progesterone, secreted by the CL (see below), prevents follicles maturing. When the CL regresses (see section 1.7) the removal of the negative feedback on the hypothalamic/pituitary axis allows the release of gonadotrophin (mainly LH) which causes maturation and ovulation of usually a single follicle. Twin or multiple ovulations are uncommon (see section 3.4) due to the secretion of local hormones such as inhibin by the dominant follicle. Various growth hormones secreted by the follicular cells also play a role in folliculogenesis.

Selection of the follicle destined for ovulation occurs about 3–4 days before ovulation (normally on day 16 or 17 of the oestrous cycle). The mature follicle is normally about 20 mm in diameter at the time of ovulation, although follicles can be capable of ovulation from about 8 mm in diameter, the size and timing being dependent upon induction of the preovulatory LH surge (see section 1.7). The anovulatory follicles regress and become atretic. At virtually any stage of the oestrous cycle, follicles up to 1.5 cm in diameter can be identified by palpation and transrectal ultrasonography in the presence of a functional CL (see sections 1.14 and 1.15).

At ovulation, the follicle ruptures through a breach in the *tunica albuginea* which surrounds the ovary. The oocyte (egg) is liberated whilst surrounded by a mass of cells – the *cumulus oophorus* (see Fig. 1.1) – and is harvested by the fimbriae of the uterine tube (oviduct) adjacent to the ovary in which ovulation has occurred.

The cavity previously occupied by the ruptured follicle is quickly invaded by the cells of the granulosal and thecal layers which become luteal cells and form the CL. The stimulus for this change is derived from LH; for some time before ovulation occurs, LH receptors have been developing in the granulosal and thecal cells. In the CL, there are two types of steroidogenic cells: the large luteal cells are derived from the granulosal cells and the small luteal cells from the thecal cells.

The CL is fully formed after about 7 days and persists in this state until about 17 days of the oestrous cycle, when it starts to regress both at a cellular level and physically.

Figure 1.2 illustrates follicular and CL development and regression during the oestrous cycle.

1.6 HORMONES PRODUCED BY THE OVARY

The developing Graafian follicle produces oestradiol-17β and two other hormones which are metabolites, i.e. oestrone and oestriol. The CL pro-

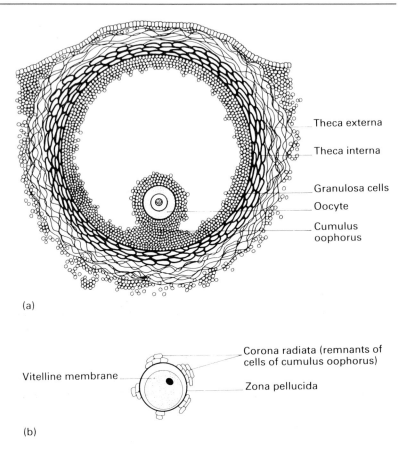

(a)

(b)

Fig. 1.1. (a) Structure of the Graafian follicle (b) Oocyte after ovulation. (Diagram (a) reproduced from Hunter, R.F.H. (1982) *Physiology and Technology of Reproduction in Female Domestic Animals.* Academic Press, London.)

duces progesterone and oxytocin, both of which play a key role in controlling ovarian cyclical activity in the cow.

1.7 HORMONAL CHANGES DURING THE OESTROUS CYCLE

Ovarian function is controlled mainly by the secretion of the hormones FSH and LH from the anterior pituitary gland. These in turn are released following the action of a polypeptide produced by the hypothalamus and transported to the anterior pituitary in the hypophyseal portal circulation. This is referred to as luteinising hormone releasing hormone (LHRH) or GnRH, since it is likely that in the cow a single substance is responsible for the release of both FSH and LH.

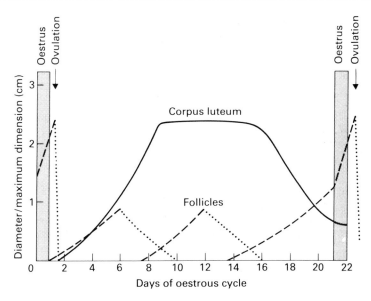

Fig. 1.2. Growth and regression of the follicles and CL during the oestrous cycle (this is an example of a cow with three waves of follicular growth).

FSH is responsible for early growth of follicles. LH causes final maturation and ovulation, and also stimulates the formation and maintenance of the CL (luteotrophic effect). These two hormones are released in surges around the time of oestrus, ovulation occurring 24–32 h after the combined FSH/LH surge.

Follicular growth and maturation results in an increase in the production of oestrogens, especially oestradiol-17β, with peak values occurring at the onset of behavioural oestrus. This stimulates the hypothalamic/pituitary axis to release the LH surge required for follicular maturation and ovulation. A second, smaller peak of oestradiol occurs 6 days after oestrus; its significance is not known.

The CL, formed from the luteinised granulosal and thecal cells, produces progesterone. This rises from basal levels 3–4 days after oestrus, reaching maximum values at about 8 days which persist until 16 or 17 days, before declining to reach basal levels at the time of next oestrus. Prolactin, another pituitary hormone, also increases around the time of oestrus, but its role at this stage is not known.

Progesterone, and hence the CL, plays a pivotal role in controlling cyclical activity since this hormone exerts a negative feedback effect upon the hypothalamic/pituitary axis, largely suppressing gonadotrophin release.

In the absence of pregnancy, the CL regresses (see section 2.9). Luteolysis, as the mechanism is called, results from the episodic release of prostaglandin F$_2\alpha$ (PGF$_2\alpha$) from the endometrium in response to the binding of oxytocin – secreted by the CL – to the oxytocin receptors on the endometrium. Oxytocin receptors start to increase in number from about days 16 and 17 of the oestrous cycle, reaching a maximum at oestrus; the development of the oxytocin receptors is under the influence of oestradiol, progesterone and oxytocin itself. The pulsatile release of $PGF_2\alpha$ starts about day 17 and increases in both frequency and amplitude. It reaches the CL directly via the ovarian artery, having passed directly from the venous drainage of the uterus.

As the CL regresses the negative feedback of progesterone on the hypothalamic/pituitary axis is removed. This is followed by a rise in FSH and LH concentrations which stimulate follicular growth and oestradiol-17β synthesis, and thus triggers the FSH/LH surge with follicular maturation, ovulation and CL formation. The hormone changes are illustrated in Fig. 1.3.

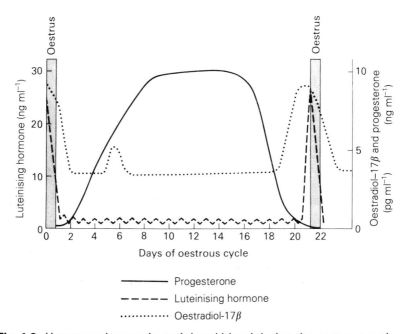

Fig. 1.3. Hormone changes in peripheral blood during the oestrous cycle.

1.8   OESTRUS AND ITS DETECTION

The average duration of oestrus is about 15 h; however, there is a wide range of 2–30 h. Once the cow has had her first ovulation postpartum it is rare for her not to show any signs of oestrus; hence 'silent heat' is a rarity.

Signs of oestrus

Signs of oestrus are many and varied:

● Increased restlessness and activity which results in grouping of sexually active individuals and depressed feeding and milk yields

- Bellowing when isolated.
- Slight increase (0.1°C) in body temperature.
- Clear vulval mucus – 'bulling string'.
- Rub marks and excoriation of the tail-head, and soiling of the flanks with mud or muck.
- Mounting other cows, particularly mounting the cow from the head-end.
- Standing to be mounted.

The only reliable signs are standing to be mounted and head-mounting (in the small percentage of cows that exhibit this). A cow might be mounted once or over a hundred times during a single oestrus; the duration of a positive mounting response should be at least 5 s.

The most important reason for poor reproductive performance is the difficulty of detecting oestrus, especially in large herds. This is due to variations between cows and because there is greater oestrous behaviour at night.

Methods of detection
Detection usually depends upon observation of a standing response when ridden. Thus for good detection there must be:

- clear identification of individual animals with freeze brands, collars and large ear tags;
- adequate lighting to aid accurate identification;
- a permanent record of the cow's identity made at the time of observation;
- a regular routine of at least three 20–30 min observation periods throughout the 24 h, at times other than milking or feeding, when the herd is not being disturbed e.g. 0800, 1400 and 2100 h, the last time being the most important;
- adequate areas with enough space and a good floor surface to enable the cows to express oestrous behaviour;
- a record of *all* oestrous periods even before the earliest service date.

1.9   AIDS TO IMPROVING OESTRUS DETECTION

- Tail paint, when applied to the base of the tail and sacrum, is removed by rubbing when a cow stands to be ridden. It is cheap and quite effective when used sensibly on a selective basis. If the paint surface becomes cracked or flakes it needs to be repaired by reapplication.
- KaMaR heat-mount detectors (see Fig. 1.4) are activated in the same way as that described for tail paint. They are more expensive than the latter and cows must be identified when they are affixed because in some cases riding displaces the device.
- Closed circuit television with time-lapse video is quite effective when used selectively, for example during the hours of night when the cows are not observed. Good cow identification is important.

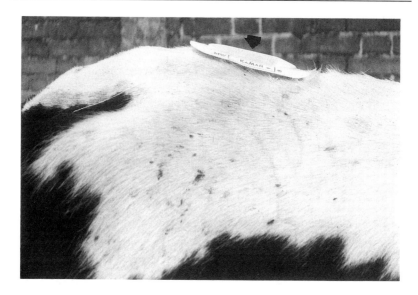

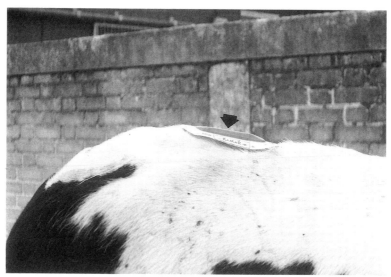

Fig. 1.4. Cow with KaMaR heat-mount detector attached to sacral region. (a) Non-activated; note white plastic dome (➥). (b) Activated; the plastic dome is now red (➥).

- Teaser bulls or androgenised cows will identify cows that are in oestrus provided that they have some form of marker, such as a chin-ball device. There are safety problems and the danger of the spread of venereal diseases with bulls. Some acquire harems of specific cows.
- Measurement of certain physiological changes, such as increased body temperature, alterations in electrical impedance within the vagina or vaginal mucus, can be used, but this requires specific equipment.

- Milk progesterone assays can predict the onset of oestrus. They can either be used routinely on alternate days from 25–30 days postpartum. Alternatively, if oestrus has been detected and the cow has been inseminated, a milk sample can be collected on day 19 after that date or on days 17, 19 and 21 or days 16, 18 and 20. A low progesterone concentration indicates that the cow is close to or in oestrus and should be subject to closer surveillance.
- It is possible to eliminate the need for oestrus detection by synchronising oestrus and ovulation, followed by fixed-time artificial insemination (AI) (see sections 1.12 and 1.13).

1.10   METHODS OF ARTIFICIALLY CONTROLLING THE OESTROUS CYCLE

In order to artificially control the oestrus cycle, the animal concerned must have reached puberty and be undergoing normal cyclical activity. There are two methods:

(1) The length of the lifespan of the CL is shortened.
(2) An exogenous source of progesterone is used to replace the function of the CL.

1.11   SHORTENING THE LIFESPAN OF THE CORPUS LUTEUM

Prostaglandin $F_{2}\alpha$ is the natural luteolysin in the cow and is responsible for its demise before the next oestrus (see section 1.7). Thus if $PGF_{2}\alpha$ or its analogues are administered parenterally to a cow with a CL it will cause premature regression and an early return to oestrus. However, the CL is unresponsive for the first 4–5 days after ovulation; furthermore, once the CL has started to regress spontaneously at day 16 or 17 this process cannot be accelerated.

1.12 PROGESTAGENS – PRINCIPLES OF USE

An exogenous source of progesterone or a synthetic progestagen functions as an artificial CL, thus exerting a negative feedback effect upon the hypothalamic/pituitary axis and suppressing cyclical activity. When this is removed, in the absence of a functional CL, there is a return to oestrus and a resumption of cyclical activity.

If, in a group of animals, progestagens are removed at the same time, there is good synchronisation provided that there is no residual endogenous progestagen derived from a CL that has outlived the duration of the implant. Thus it is necessary to induce luteolysis or suppress the formation of a CL.

Synchronisation with a progesterone-releasing intravaginal device (PRID)

The progesterone-releasing intravaginal device (PRID) is a stainless steel flat coil covered with an inert elastomer incorporating 1.55 g progesterone together with a 10 mg oestradiol benzoate capsule (see Fig. 1.5).

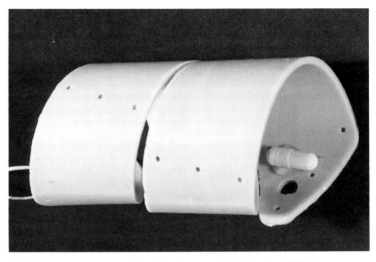

Fig. 1.5. A progesterone-releasing intravaginal device (PRID).

- The cow or heifer must not be pregnant, must not have calved within the last 20 days or have any infection of the genital tract, and must be in good bodily condition.
- Using a gentle and clean technique the PRID is inserted into the anterior vagina.
- After about 12 days it is withdrawn and oestrus occurs 2–3 days later. Fixed-time AI can be used at 48 and 72 h, or once only at 56 h, after removal.
- Animals showing behavioural oestrus several days after the removal of the PRID should be inseminated as normal.

The degree of synchronisation can be variable because oestradiol benzoate is a poor luteolytic and antiluteotrophic agent. Better results can be obtained if $PGF_2\alpha$ is injected 24 h before the PRID is removed, together with a shorter period of retention such as 8 days.

Some animals will expel the PRID and in many there is vaginal discharge which is resolved spontaneously after withdrawal; treatment is unnecessary.

Synchronisation with an intravaginal progesterone-releasing device (CIDR)

This is a Y-shaped device comprising a nylon spine covered with an elastomer containing 1.9 g progesterone; a plastic tab enables its withdrawal (see Fig. 1.6).

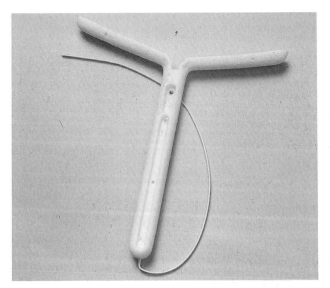

Fig. 1.6. Intravaginal progesterone-releasing device (CIDR).

The requirements are similar to those listed for the PRID except that in the absence of an oestradiol capsule $PGF_2\alpha$ must always be used. The following protocol should be followed:

- Using a clean and gentle technique, insert the CIDR into the vagina using the manufacturer's applicator.
- After 7–12 days, the CIDR should be removed by pulling gently on the plastic tab.
- A luteolytic dose of $PGF_2\alpha$ or analogue should be administered on the day of withdrawal or at any time from 6 days after insertion.
- Oestrus should occur 48–96 h after removal with cows being inseminated at the normal time, or after a fixed time of 56 h.

Synchronisation with Norgestamet

Norgestamet is a potent synthetic progestagen which is available as a subcutaneous polymer implant containing 3 mg of the active substance.

- It can be used in beef and dairy heifers and suckler cows only. Milk must not be used for human consumption.

- The cow must be at least 45 days postpartum.
- The cow or heifer must not be pregnant and must be in good bodily condition.
- The implant of 3 mg Norgestamet is inserted subcutaneously at the base of the ear and immediately afterwards 3 mg Norgestamet and 5 mg oestradiol valerate (2 ml) are injected intramuscularly.
- Nine to ten days later the implant is removed.
- Oestrus occurs 2–3 days later and fixed-time AI can be used at 48 and 72 h or once only at 56 hours, after implant removal.

Better synchronisation can be achieved if $PGF_2\alpha$ is injected 24 h before removal of the implant as oestradiol valerate is poorly luteolytic, especially early in dioestrus.

1.13   SYNCHRONISATION OF OESTRUS WITH $PGF_2\alpha$ OR ANALOGUES

To achieve synchronisation $PGF_2\alpha$ or analogue must be injected in two separate doses, 11 days apart. At the time of the second injection there will be a CL that is responsive to its luteolytic effect, resulting in oestrus 2–5 days later.

Before starting the synchronisation procedure:

- Check the physical condition of the animals, especially in the case of heifers; the latter should be in good bodily condition growing at a rate of 0.7 kg per day.
- Ensure that there are no pregnant animals and, in the case of heifers, that there is a normal genital tract on rectal palpation.
- Inform the local AI centre of the proposed dates for AI to ensure that there is adequate semen and staff available.

Then:

- Inject all of the animals with $PGF_2\alpha$ or analogue (PG_1).
- Repeat 11 days after PG_1 (PG_2).
- Use fixed-time AI at 72–84 h after PG_2, or two inseminations at 72 and 96 h or 72 and 90 h after PG_2 (recommendations vary between manufacturers).
- AI any animals that are seen in standing oestrus 5–6 days after PG_2.

Synchronisation will be much better in heifers than in cows.

Reasons for poor synchronisation

- Poor injection technique if $PGF_2\alpha$ is deposited in fat or a large volume of the injection escapes (unlikely).
- A proportion of the animals are acyclic.
- There is a delay in the formation of a CL that will respond to $PGF_2\alpha$.

This is most likely to occur in cows where progesterone concentrations remain low for a long period after ovulation (long–low progesterone).

Reasons for poor conception rates (pregnancy rates)

- Poor nutrition, especially in heifers and high yielding cows.
- Stress associated with handling and mixing different groups of animals.
- Synchronisation of recently purchased animals because they will have been stressed by the move.
- Inseminator fatigue.

A compromise regimen

Better conception rates can frequently be obtained, especially if there is good and accurate oestrus detection, if the following compromise regimen is used:

- Inject all animals with $PGF_2\alpha$ or analogues (PG_1).
- Observe for signs of oestrus and inseminate any cows or heifers as normal.
- Animals that have not been observed in oestrus after 11 days are injected with a second dose of $PGF_2\alpha$ or analogues (PG_2).
- Fixed-time insemination as described in section 1.3.

This regimen also reduces the amount of animal handling and the quantity of prostaglandin used.

Prostaglandins and analogues available for cattle

- Dinoprost. Synthetic naturally occurring $PGF_2\alpha$, dose rate 25 mg.
- Cloprostenol. Synthetic analogue, dose rate 500 μg.
- Luprostiol. Dose rate 15 mg for cows and 7.5 mg for heifers.

1.14 CLINICAL EXAMINATION OF THE GENITAL SYSTEM

The genital system can be examined by rectal palpation and β mode ultrasonography using the transrectal approach. The vestibule, vagina and external opening of the cervix can be examined by manual palpation or, visually, with the aid of the speculum. Before embarking upon these procedures a careful inspection of the vulva, perineum and body surfaces is important.

External clinical examination

- Examine the base of the tail (tail-head) for ruffled hair or abrasions that suggest that the cow may have been standing to be ridden by other cows and hence has been in oestrus.
- Examine the flanks for signs of muddy or mucky hoof marks indicative of being ridden by other cows.

- Examine the perineum and tail for signs of discharge. This could be a normal, physiological discharge associated with oestrus, metoestrus or postpartum lochia (see section 5.6), or it might be pathological, associated with an inflammatory exudate or pus.
- Examine the vulva for evidence of fresh or healed injuries. Part the labia and examine the mucosa for general colour and the presence of papules, pustules, vesicles, ulcers or raised granulomatous lesions.
- Examine the mammary gland to determine the stage of lactation.
- Examine the pelvis and pelvic ligaments to determine the degree of relaxation in the cow approaching calving.

Vaginal examination using a speculum

When a speculum is used it must be sterile for each cow or, alternatively, a sterile speculum guard tube can be used with certain types (see Fig. 1.7), these usually have their own light source. The conventional speculum requires a torch or other hand-held light source to be available.

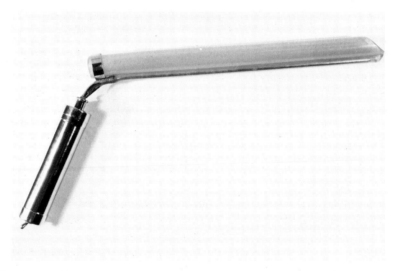

Fig. 1.7. A vaginal speculum.

The procedure for using a self-illuminating speculum is as follows:

- Clean the vulva thoroughly.
- Part the labia and gently insert the lubricated speculum at an angle of about 30° from the horizontal plane upwards into the vestibule and then horizontally over the pelvic floor.
- As the speculum is inserted note the colour and appearance of the vaginal mucosa and fluid as well as any aberrant structures.
- Note the colour, shape and degree of dilatation of the external opening

of the cervix, as well as the presence and appearance of any fluid that escapes from the cervical canal.

- Note the appearance of any fluid that pools in the anterior vagina.

Manual examination of the vagina

This is not possible in a nulliparous heifer.

- Gently insert a clean, lubricated, gloved hand into the vagina.
- Note evidence of strictures, abscesses and other abnormalities.
- Palpate the cervix for evidence of tears, lesions and the degree of dilatation of the external opening.
- Scoop any pooled fluid present on the floor of the anterior vagina into the palm of the hand and examine when withdrawn; note the presence of a urine pool.

Rectal palpation

A regular routine is required and the vulva should be observed for evidence of secretions or discharges throughout the procedure.

The *vagina* is difficult to identify because it has a flaccid, thin wall, unless a previous vaginal examination has resulted in the formation of a temporary pneumovagina when it will be distended.

The *cervix* is an important landmark. Note its position relative to the brim of the pelvis, its size and shape and the degree of mobility. In non-pregnant heifers the cervix is about 2–3 cm in diameter and 5–6 cm in length. During pregnancy it becomes enlarged and although it regresses postpartum the overall size increases with successive pregnancies. In old pluriparous cows it is 5–6 cm in diameter and up to 10 cm in length. The cervix tapers slightly cranially and it is frequently possible to palpate the annular folds. Abscesses associated with calving or AI injuries cause marked distortion.

The cervix in the heifer is always intrapelvic whilst in normal, non-pregnant parous animals it is located on the brim of the pelvis or just over. With advancing pregnancy it is pulled further over the brim.

In the normal, non-pregnant animal it is freely mobile laterally and cranio-caudally. As pregnancy advances the pull of the gravid uterus reduces the mobility, as do such pathological conditions as adhesions, pyometra and tumours.

The *bifurcation of the uterine horns* can be identified just cranial to the cervix, especially if they are compressed against the pelvic brim, as a fissure or cleft before the horns diverge (see Fig. 1.8).

The *uterine horns* initially curve downwards and forwards and then backwards and upwards towards the tip which is situated 5–6 cm from the cervix (see Fig. 1.8). The size of the horns will depend upon whether or not the animal is pregnant and the stage of pregnancy, postpartum or suffering from some pathological condition.

The horns of the non-gravid uterus are about 35–40 cm in length and 4–

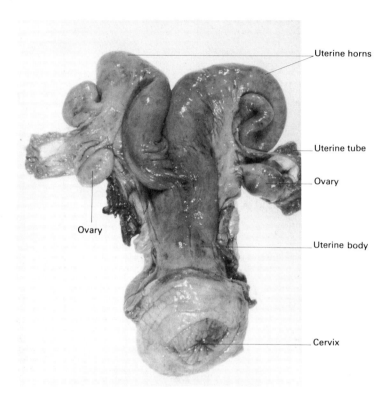

Uterine horns

Uterine tube

Ovary

Ovary

Uterine body

Cervix

Fig. 1.8. Genital tract of the cow.

5 cm in diameter; they are more or less equal in size. In pregnancy (see section 2.11) and immediately postpartum (see section 5.5) there is disparity. With each successive pregnancy they become slightly enlarged.

The *uterine horns undergo cyclical changes* which can be identified on palpation. During dioestrus they are flaccid, and it is difficult to identify their outline along the entire length of the horn. As the CL regresses and there is follicular growth 1–2 days before oestrus, the tone in the uterus increases so that the horns become turgid and coiled, especially when manipulated. The tone increases during oestrus and, although it does decline after oestrus and ovulation, it persists for a further 1–2 days.

Uterine tubes (Fallopian tubes or oviducts) are convoluted structures about 20–25 cm in length (see Fig. 1.9). When they are normal they are difficult to identify on palpation; hence, if identification is easy it usually suggests that they are thickened or enlarged (see Fig. 7.3).

The *ovarian bursa* is difficult to palpate per rectum. It should be free from the surface of the ovary (see Fig. 1.10).

The *ovaries* are best located by following the uterine horns around to the greater curvature and then gently sweeping back towards the cervix with

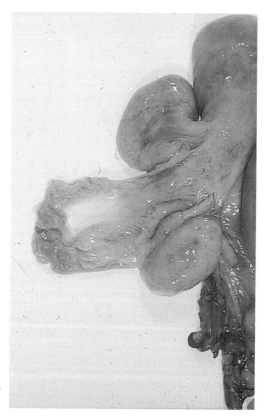

Fig. 1.9. Ovary and normal, convoluted uterine tube.

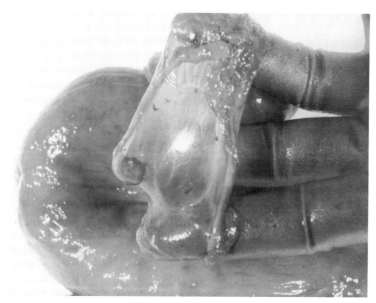

Fig. 1.10. Ovarian bursa.

the tips of the fingers. Alternatively, on locating the cervix and bifurcation the fingers can be swept downwards or either side towards the pelvic floor and brim. In heifers the ovaries are usually intrapelvic, whilst in pluriparous cows they are usually located just on or over the brim of the pelvis. With advancing pregnancy they are pulled down into the abdomen, eventually becoming out of reach.

On palpation of the ovaries their position, size and the nature of the structures present on the ovaries should be assessed. The structures that are palpable are: follicles, luteinised follicles, corpora lutea, cysts and corpora albicantes.

Follicles vary in size, reaching a maximum of 2–2.5 cm in diameter. They are fluid-filled and hence fluctuate on palpation. The ease of identification will depend upon their size, position on the ovary and the presence of other structures. Follicular growth occurs throughout the oestrous cycle and follicles are frequently as large as 1.3–1.5 cm diameter in mid-dioestrus associated with a mature CL (see Fig. 1.11). Identification of a follicle in the ovary of a cow is of little value as the sole method of assessing the stage of the oestrous cycle.

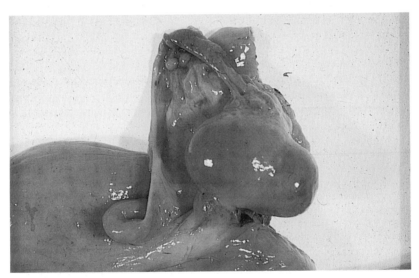

Fig. 1.11. Ovary containing mature CL and mid-dioestrus follicle.

Luteinised follicles are not common, occurring most frequently in the immediate postpartum period before normal cyclical activity has been established (see section 5.1); they arise from the luteinisation of an anovulatory follicle. Identification on rectal palpation is difficult. They are about 2–2.5 cm in diameter with a slightly thicker wall than a normal follicle. They function similarly to a CL although their lifespan is probably shorter.

The *corpus luteum* forms as a sequel to ovulation; thus if it is palpated the only immediate assumption that can be made is that the cow has ovulated at some stage. The CL may be associated with dioestrus, pregnancy or occasionally it may be persistent, associated with pyometra (see sections 7.6 and 11.10).

Positive identification of a CL is not always possible, however, since the mature CL is the structure that results in normal, physiological enlargement of the ovary; its presence can sometimes be assumed. Confirmation can be made by the presence of elevated milk or plasma progesterone concentrations or by transrectal ultrasonography (see Figs 1.16f to h).

The age of the CL can be assessed by its size and consistency although both methods can be inaccurate. Immediately after ovulation it is usually possible to palpate a sight depression at the site of ovulation; there will also be marked uterine tone (see Table 1.1). As the CL grows, the ovary enlarges and the CL usually starts to protrude from the surface of the ovary; it is soft and yielding on palpation. It reaches its maximum size of about 2.5–3 cm in diameter 7–8 days after oestrus and remains so until days 16–17 when it starts to shrink and become harder; at the same time there is increased uterine tone (Table 1.1). During the 7–17 days of the cycle, changes in ovarian size are due to follicular growth and regression (see Figs 1.12; 1.13).

A significant proportion of CLs have a central fluid-filled cavity or vacuole; such structures are normal (see Fig 1.14 and Figs 1.16g and h).

The ease and accuracy of palpation of a CL depends upon its degree of protrusion and its shape.

Table 1.1. Changes in the ovary and tubular genital tract during the oestrus cycle.

Day of cycle	Ovary	Uterus	Vaginal discharge
0 (oestrus)	Regressing CL <1 cm, perhaps follicles 1 cm	Marked tone, coiled horns increased on palpation	Copious, clear, elastic mucus
1 (ovulation)	Regressing CL <1 cm, soft ovulation depression	Good tone, coiled horns	Some clear or cloudy mucus
3	Developing soft CL 1–1.5 cm diameter	Slight tone	Bright red, blood-stained, cloudy mucus
7–17	Fully formed CL 2.5–3 cm diameter Follicles up to 1 cm diameter	Flaccid uterus	No discharge
17–19	Hard, regressing CL <1.5 cm diameter	Moderate to good tone	No discharge
21	As for day 0		

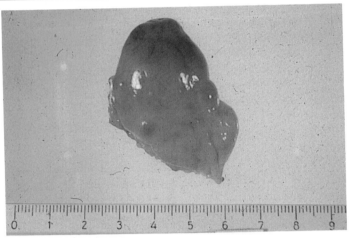

Fig. 1.12. Ovary containing mature CL.

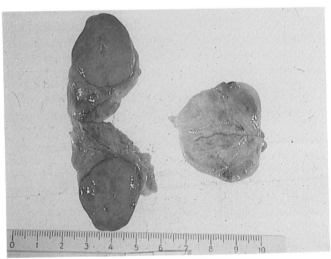

Fig. 1.13. Sectioned paired ovaries from a cow in mid-dioestrus. Left ovary contains a fully formed, mature CL; the right ovary has a small follicle and the remains of the regressed CL of the previous cycle.

Cysts are fluid-filled structures >2.5 cm in diameter, persisting and usually associated with aberrant reproductive behaviour (see sections 7.6 and 7.8 and Figs 1.16i and j).

Corpora albicantes are raised, white structures, the remnants of the corpora lutea of pregnancies. They persist throughout the life of the cow and in old pluriparous animals give a 'gritty' texture to the ovary.

The changes in the genital tract during the oestrous cycle are shown in Table 1.1.

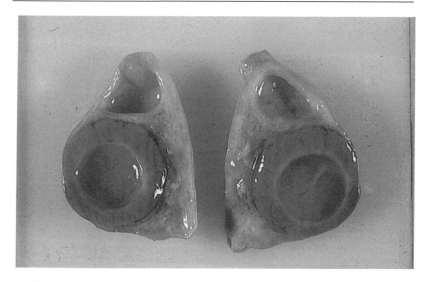

Fig. 1.14. Section of ovary from a cow in mid-dioestrus. Note the vacuolated CL and small, mid-dioestrus follicle.

1.15 ULTRASONOGRAPHY

Principle

The genital system of the cow can be examined using transrectal B-(brightness) mode ultrasonography; an example of the type of equipment that can be used is shown in Fig. 1.15.

- The source of the high frequency sound waves are the piezo crystals present in the transducer probe (in the type shown in Fig 1.15 they are present in parallel rows, hence the term 'linear array').
- The sound waves impinge upon the tissues and are reflected back to the transducer probe resulting in the formation of an image which is displayed on the screen.
- Fluid-filled structures such as follicles, cysts and fetal sacs poorly reflect the sound waves and are referred to as anechogenic or non-echogenic, whereas solid tissues such as bone or muscle readily reflect them (up to 99%) and are referred to as hyperechogenic. An anechoic structure appears black and a hyperechoic structure white, with other tissues producing varying shades of grey.
- The different degrees of reflection result in a moving (real-time), two-dimensional image appearing on the screen, the imaged tissue being in the shape of a rectangle.
- Several types of transducers are generally used for transrectal ultrasonography in the cow; a 5 MHz gives better tissue penetration but poorer resolution than a 7.5 MHz transducer.

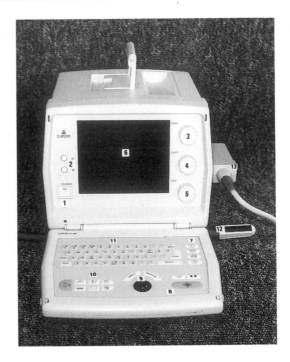

Key

1 On/off
2 Monitor controls   Brightness/contrast of the screen is independent of printer
3 Overall gain   Sensitivity of probe to returning echos
4 Near gain   Balance sensitivity of probe to superficial echos
5 Far gain   Balance sensitivity of probe to deep echos
6 Screen   Landscape presentation allows both linear and sector images
7 Screen mode   Splitting and motion mode
8 Freeze   Often supplemented with cable connected pedal
9 Measurement   Follicle diameters, wall thickness, area calculations
10 Processing mode   Adjust grey scales, edge enhancement, frame speed
11 Keyboard   Enter names, notes, diagnoses
12 Probe   3–7.5 MHz, linear or sector according to application
13 Probe connector

Fig. 1.15. Portable B-mode ultrasound scanner. (Courtesy of Stephen Constable, BCF Technology Ltd.)

Technique

Using the B-mode ultrasound to image the genital system of the cow requires practice, patience and care so that the rectal mucosa is not damaged.

- Evacuate faeces from the rectum.
- Apply plenty of cellulose-based obstetrical lubricant to a gloved hand and the surface of the transducer probe.
- Grasp the transducer probe in the palm of the hand between the thumb and fourth finger and gently insert it into the rectum; it may be necessary to use the other hand to feed in the cable.

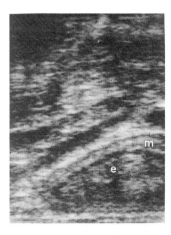

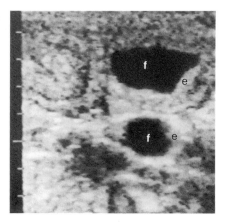

Fig. 1.16a. Transverse section of non-gravid uterine horn showing endometrium (e) and muscularis (m).

Fig. 1.16b. Transverse section of gravid horn at 25 days of gestation showing two sections of coiled horn containing allantoic fluid (f) and endometrium (e).

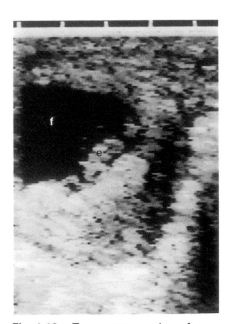

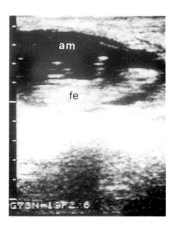

Fig. 1.16c. Transverse section of gravid horn at 35 days of gestation showing embryo (e) surrounded by fetal fluid (f). (Scale: 6.5 mm.)

Fig. 1.16d. Transverse section of gravid horn at 55 days of gestation showing fetus (fe) surrounded by amniotic fluid (am). (Scale: 6.5 mm.)

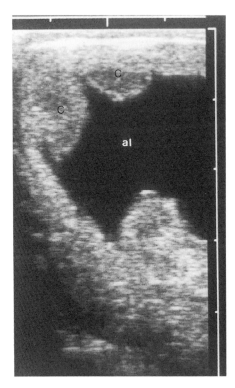

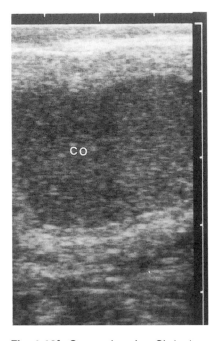

Fig. 1.16f. Ovary showing CL (co) which has a distinctive 'speckled' echotexture and defined border from the rest of the ovarian stroma. (Scale: 6 mm.)

Fig. 1.16e. Transverse section of gravid horn in mid-gestation showing caruncles/cotyledons (c) and allantoic fluid (al). (Scale: 6 mm.)

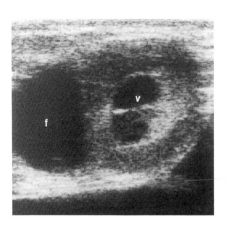

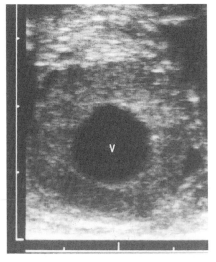

Fig. 1.16g. Ovary with CL with central vacuole (v) and mid-cycle follicle (f). (Scale: 6.5 mm.)

Fig. 1.16h. Ovary with CL with central vacuole (v). (Scale: 6.5 mm.)

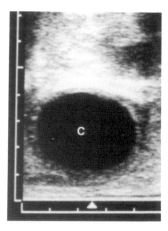

Fig. 1.16i. Ovary with follicular cyst (c) >3 cm in diameter. (Scale: 6.5 mm.)

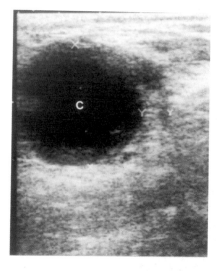

Fig. 1.16j. (above) Ovary with luteal cyst (c) >3 cm in diameter, not thick wall (x – y).

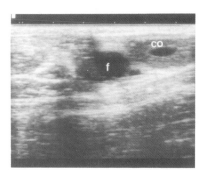

Fig. 1.16k. (left) Ovary with vacuolated CL (co) and follicle (f). (Scale: 6.5 mm.)

(All parts of Fig. 1.16(a–k) are courtesy of Stephen Constable, BCF Technology Ltd.)

Identify the structures with the thumb and fourth finger whilst gently pressing the transducer so that it is in close contact with the rectal wall adjacent to the structure.

- Use a regular routine, imaging cervix, uterine horns and ovaries in that order.
- The cervix and ovaries can be imaged most readily in a longitudinal plane whilst the horns, because they are coiled, cannot be imaged along their length but are best done transversely. In order to identify the whole structure, it is necessary to gently rotate the transducer about its longitudinal axis.

Identification of structures

Figure 1.16a–k shows the appearance of the structures most readily identified.

2 Normal Pregnancy

2.1 OVULATION

The ovulated oocyte enters the fimbria of the adjacent uterine tube which is
closely apposed to the surface of the ovary during, and after, oestrus. The
oocyte is transported by the action of cilia and peristaltic contractions and
perhaps tubal secretions to the ampulla where fertilisation occurs (see Fig.
2.1). Delayed or premature transport can affect its viability. The oocyte is
capable of being fertilised for 8–12 h after ovulation although best results
are obtained within 6 h.

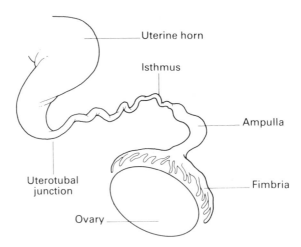

Fig. 2.1. The uterine (Fallopian) tube.

2.2 FERTILISATION

Whilst small numbers of sperm will have reached the uterine tube within 15
min of mating or AI, at least 6–8 h are required after natural mating before
a sufficiently large number of sperm is present in the uterine tube to ensure
a good fertilisation rate. This is probably slightly shorter when sperm are
deposited in the uterus at AI.

Spermatozoa undergo maturation processes before they are capable of fertilisation. These processes are called capacitation and the acrosome reaction; these are stimulated by the uterine secretions and follicular fluid. The time required is 4 h. Sperm retain their motility for 15–56 h. Although they are fertile for up to 30–48 h, there is some decline in fertility after 15–20 h.

When a sperm has penetrated the zona pellucida (see Fig. 1.1), others are generally prevented from doing so by the vitelline block. When several sperm penetrate the oocyte it is called polyspermy and the developing embryos will die.

2.3 EMBRYONIC DEVELOPMENT

See Table 2.1 below.

After the organ systems are formed (organogenesis is complete) the calf is now considered to be a fetus.

Table 2.1 Development of the embryo

Days after ovulation		Growth of embryo
0–1		1 cell
1–2	Uterine tube	2 cells
1–2		4 cells
2–3		8 cells
3–6	Enters uterus	Morula
6–9		Blastocyst
8–10		Hatching blastocyst
12–14		Elongation of blastocyst
13–16		Amnion formed
20–28		First changes in trophoblast adjacent to uterine caruncles
24–28		Allantois fully formed
35		Allantois fills and distends gravid horn
45		Organogenesis complete

2.4 FETAL MEMBRANES

Amnion forms from about 13–16 days after fertilisation as an outfolding from the ectodermic vesicle. It becomes a double-walled sac which completely surrounds the embryo/fetus except at the umbilical ring (see Fig. 2.2). The amnion is a fairly tough transparent membrane.

Allantois arises 14–21 days after fertilisation as an outgrowth from the embryonic hind gut. The outer part fuses with the chorionic trophoblast to form the allantochorion, which is a highly vascular structure and is involved

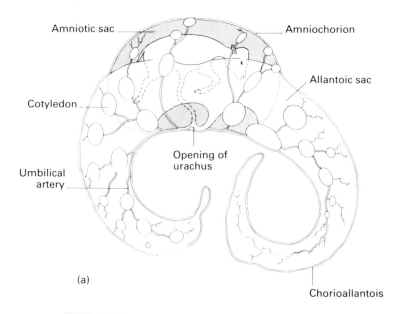

Amniotic sac

Amniochorion

Allantoic sac

Cotyledon

Umbilical
artery

Opening of
urachus

(a)

Chorioallantois

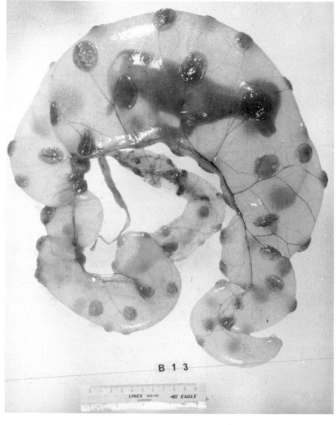

B 1 3

(b)

Fig. 2.2. (a) and (b) Fetal membranes of the calf, showing the cotyledons.
(Diagram (a) reproduced from Steven, D.H. (1982) Placentation in the mare.
Journal of Reproduction and Fertility, Suppl. 31, 41–5.)

in the formation of the placenta. The inner part lies over the amnion (See Fig. 2.2).

2.5 FETAL FLUIDS

The amnion surrounds the amniotic fluid which protects the embryo/fetus from mechanical injury and possibly infection, and provides a vehicle for excretion. Towards the end of gestation it becomes viscous, acting as a lubricant at calving and facilitating the expulsion of the calf.

The allantoic fluid is watery. It protects the embryo/fetus from mechanical trauma and provides a space for the deposition of fetal urine via the urachus.

The approximate volumes of the fetal fluids during pregnancy are given in Table 2.2.

Table 2.2 Approximate volumes of fetal fluids during pregnancy

Stage of pregnancy (days)	Amniotic fluid (ml)	Allantoic fluid (ml)
30	0.5	55
35–45	21	140
46–60	96	202
61–90	375	415
91–120	1450	1170
121–150	3026	1417
151–180	2544	2638
181–210	1541	4672
211–240	2028	4893
241–Term	2272	9862

The total volume of fetal fluids increases progressively throughout pregnancy with a rapid rise at 70–80 days. During the first third of gestation the volume of allantoic is greater than amniotic; during the second third the volume of amniotic is greater than allantoic; whilst during the last third the volume of allantoic fluid is greater than the amniotic. There are considerable variations in the volumes of fluid associated with individual fetuses of the same gestational age.

2.6 FETAL GROWTH AND CROWN–RUMP LENGTHS

The average weights of embryonic/fetal singleton calves are shown in Table 2.3.

Table 2.3 Average weights of embryonic/fetal singleton calves*

Stage of gestation (days)	‚Embryonic/fetal weight	Crown–rump length (cm)
30	0.3–0.5 g	0.8–1
40	1–1.5 g	1.75–2.5
50	3–6 g	3.5–5.5
60	8–30 g	6–8
70	25–100 g	7–10
80	120–200 g	8–13
90	200–400 g	13–17
120	1–2 kg	22–32
150	3–4 kg	30–45
180	5–10 kg	40–60
210	8–18 kg	55–75
240	15–25 kg	60–85
270	20–50 kg	70–100

* Twin calves will be relatively smaller and there will be considerable individual and breed variations in singleton calves. See section 3.4 Twinning and multiples and section 3.5 Freemartins.

2.7 ESTIMATION OF FETAL AGE

Several formulae have been derived in estimating fetal age, provided that the crown–rump length (CRL) is measured.

$$\textit{Formula for estimating fetal age in days} = 2.5 \times (\text{CRL cm} + 21)$$
$$\text{Thus if CRL} = 10 \text{ cm}$$
$$\text{fetal age in days} = 2.5 \times (10 + 21)$$
$$= 2.5 \times 31$$
$$= 77.5 \text{ days}$$

or, less accurately,

$$\textit{Formula for estimating fetal age in months} = \sqrt{2 \times \text{CRL inches}}$$
$$\text{Thus if CRL} = 4.5 \text{ inches}$$
$$\text{fetal age} = \sqrt{2 \times 4.5}$$
$$= \sqrt{9}$$
$$= 3 \text{ months}$$

2.8 PLACENTA

The placenta of the cow is referred to as a cotyledonary or multiplex placenta because it is confined to well-defined restricted oval or circular areas of the allantochorion – the cotyledons (see Fig. 2.2b). These develop in those parts that are adjacent to the specialised areas of the endometrium – the caruncles.

The placenta can also be categorised according to the microscopic structure and in particular the number of tissue layers which separate maternal and fetal circulations – it is usually referred to as epithelialchorial. However, synepithelialchorial is a more appropriate terminology because of the initial fetomaternally-derived syncitium lining the endometrium and the continual migration and fusion of chorionic cells during pregnancy. The interface between fetal and maternally-derived tissues comprises inter-digitating chorionic villi and caruncular crypts. In addition, there are microvilli on the surfaces of the apposed epithelial cells held together by an adhesive protein referred to as the 'glue line'.

2.9 MATERNAL RECOGNITION OF PREGNANCY

If a cow is not pregnant she will return to oestrus at the normal inter-oestrous interval (18–24 days) after service or AI (see section 1.3). If fer-tilisation occurs with subsequent embryonic development then the CL will persist and there will be no return to oestrus. This phenomenon is referred to as 'the maternal recognition of pregnancy' which occurs from about 14 days after oestrus and insemination. The trophoblast of the developing embryo secretes a protein which is a type 1 interferon and is referred to as tau or IFNΥ. It maintains early pregnancy by sustaining the inhibitory effect on CL-derived oxytocin until its stores have been depleted by about 20 days, thereby preventing regression of the CL (see section 1.7). IFNΥ secretion reaches a maximum at between 16 and 19 days and persists for up to 38 days.

2.10 ENDOCRINOLOGY OF PREGNANCY

The most important hormone is progesterone, which suppresses normal cyclical activity via its negative feedback effect upon the anterior pituitary (see section 1.7). Progesterone also stimulates changes in the endome-trium that are conducive to the nourishment and development of the embryo. Towards the end of pregnancy there is a decline in progesterone (see Fig. 2.3).

Progesterone is synthesised by the CL, the feto-placental unit and the adrenocortex. After about 150 days of gestation the CL is not necessary for the maintenance of pregnancy because it is no longer the major source of this hormone.

2.11 METHODS OF PREGNANCY DIAGNOSIS

It is the early detection of the non-pregnant cow that is important in the reproductive management of individual animals.

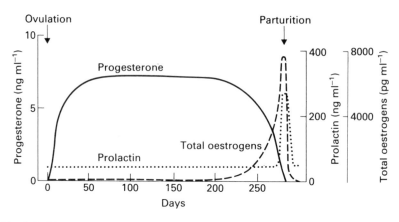

Fig. 2.3. Hormone concentration in the peripheral circulation of the cow during pregnancy and at parturition. (Reproduced from Arthur, G.H., Noakes, D.E. & Pearson, H. (1982) *Veterinary Reproduction and Obstetrics*, 5th edn Baillière Tindall, Eastbourne.)

Early detection of pregnancy will be followed by embryonic or fetal death in some individuals resulting in false negatives (see sections 2.12 and 7.3)

(1) *18–24 days.* Failure to return to oestrus which is dependent upon the detection of oestrus (see sections 1.8 and 1.9). Some cows show oestrus during pregnancy, especially later on.

(2) *18–24 days.* Persistence of a CL on rectal palpation. It is not possible to distinguish between a CL or dioestrus and pregnancy.

(3) *Measurement of plasma or milk progesterone concentrations* by radioimmunoassay, or ELISA (enzyme-linked immunosorbent assay). Milk concentrations closely follow the changes that occur in plasma although absolute values are higher (see Fig. 2.4) because progesterone is soluble in milk fat.

Milk assay is usually performed on a well-mixed bulk sample from the individual cow, although fore-milk and strippings can be used, collected 24 days after service or AI. If a preservative tablet containing potassium dichromate and mercuric chloride is added to the sample it can be retained at room temperature for several months without any significant loss of progesterone.

Milk progesterone assay is about 85% accurate for positive diagnosis of pregnancy and almost 100% accurate for identifying the non-pregnant cow. The accuracy can be improved if a milk sample is collected on the day of AI; a low milk progesterone concentration will confirm that the cow is not in dioestrus and is probably in oestrus.

Reasons for false positives:

• Incorrect timing of AI when the cow is inseminated in dioestrus (see Fig. 2.4).

• Prenatal death after the sample has been collected.

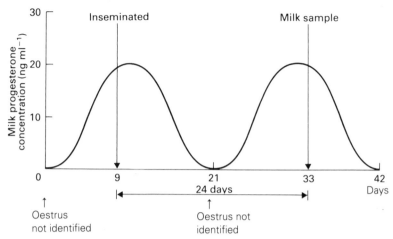

Fig. 2.4. Progesterone concentrations in the milk during the oestrous cycle to show a false positive for pregnancy due to mistimed AI.

- Luteal cyst (see section 7.6).
- Persistent CL associated with chronic uterine infection (see sections 11.9 and 11.10).
- Shorter-than-average interval between two successive oestruses.

Reasons for false negatives:

- Inadequate mixing of bulk milk sample.
- Exposure of sample to excessive heat or u.v. light.
- Incorrect identification of animal or sample.

(4) *Measurement of pregnancy-specific protein B (PSPB).* This protein is secreted by the trophoblastic ectoderm; its presence confirms pregnancy when first identified at about 24 days after service or AI.

(5) Transrectal ultrasonography at *28 days*. Although experienced persons can detect pregnancy as early as 12–14 days, for routine use 28–30 days of gestation is generally recommended to provide a high level of accuracy (see Fig. 1.16c).

(6) *30 days*. The amniotic vesicle can be palpated as a small, turgid 'pea-size' object 1 cm in diameter at 30 days by gently squeezing the uterine horns between thumb and fingers. At 35 days it is 1.7 cm in diameter. There is danger of trauma to the embryonic heart.

(7) *30–35 days*. There is some disparity in the size of the uterine horns, the one adjacent to the ovary with the CL becoming larger. There is evidence of the fluctuation of the slightly distended horn because of the presence of allantoic fluid (see section 2.5) and thinning of the uterine wall.

(8) *35–40 days*. It is possible to palpate the allantochorion at this stage (see section 2.4) using the technique of 'membrane slip'. The uterine horn is gently grasped between thumb and forefinger and then

squeezed so that the contents of the horn are allowed to slip away. The first structure to be released from grasp is the thin allantochorion before the rather thicker uterine wall.

(9) *45–50 days*. It is frequently possible to palpate the fetus at this stage as a structure rather like a piece of cork floating in fluid.

(10) *70–80 days*. The enlarged caruncles/cotyledons can be palpated from this stage as small irregularities in the wall of the uterine body and base of the horns. They become larger and more distinct with advancing pregnancy (see Fig. 1.16e).

(11) *90–120 days*. It is possible to identify a change in the pulse character of the middle uterine artery which causes it to 'buzz' or vibrate. It is referred to as fremitus. Initially it is in the artery supplying the gravid horn, subsequently it involves both.

(12) *105 days*. The identification of the conjugated hormone oestrone sulphate in milk or blood samples at this stage of gestation and later is diagnostic of pregnancy.

2.12 ACCURACY OF PREGNANCY DIAGNOSIS BY RECTAL PALPATION

Rectal palpation should be over 95% accurate provided that at least one positive sign is identified.

False positives occur because:

- The uterus is not retracted to enable detailed palpation.
- The uterus is not completely involuted (see section 5.5).
- There is pyometra (see section 11.10).
- There is mucometra.
- There is subsequent prenatal death.

False negatives occur because:

- The uterus is not retracted to enable detailed palpation.
- The recorded service date was incorrect.
- The cow has been served or inseminated since the recorded date.

3   Normal Parturition

3.1   DURATION OF PREGNANCY

The average duration of pregnancy is 280 days; however, there are considerable breed differences (see Table 3.1). The influence of genotype is seen when certain breeds of sires are crossed with cows of a different breed, with the length of gestation being extended.

Table 3.1 Gestation length and birth weights of different breeds of cattle

Breed	Average length of gestation (days) (Range given in brackets)	Average birth weight (kg)
Aberdeen Angus	280 (273–283)	28
Ayrshire	279 (277–284)	34
Brown Swiss	286 (285–287)	43.5
Charolais	287 (285–288)	43.5
Friesian/Holstein	279 (272–284)	41
Guernsey	284 (281–286)	30
Hereford	286 (280–289)	32
Jersey	280 (277–284)	24.5
Simmental	288 (285–291)	43
South Devon	287 (286–287)	44.5

Male calves have a slightly longer gestation than female calves of the same breed (1 or 2 days).

3.2   BIRTH WEIGHT

The average figures are shown for different breeds in Table 3.1. The following factors can influence birth weight:

- Genotype.
- Gestation length – larger calves from longer gestations.
- Parity of dam – smaller calves from heifers.

- Season of year.
- Nutrition – only with severe underfeeding of the dam.
- Twins or multiples.

3.3   FETAL GROWTH RATE

The period of most rapid growth rate occurs around 230 days of gestation with the fetal calf gaining weight at about 0.25 kg per day; thereafter it declines (see section 2.6).

3.4   TWINNING AND MULTIPLES

Twins occur in 1–2% of births and triplets in 0.013% of births. There is considerable breed variation and a tendency for the likelihood to increase with the advancing age of the cow. The ovulation rate, and hence the incidence of twinning or multiples, cannot be influenced by nutrition. The incidence of twin ovulation is higher than that of twin births because of the embryonic death of one of the twins.

3.5   FREEMARTINS

Freemartins normally occur when a heifer calf is born as a co-twin to a male calf. This is due to placental fusion at about 40 days of gestation. Ninety per cent of such heifer calves are freemartins. However, it is also possible to have single-born freemartins where the male fetus dies and is resorbed after placental fusion has occurred.

Diagnosis of freemartins

At birth the use of a blunt vaginal probe, such as a thermometer case, will provide good evidence, especially if the depth to which the probe will enter the vagina unimpeded is compared with a normal heifer calf of similar age. It is usually about one-third of the depth of the normal calf, i.e. about 3–5 cm. Accurate confirmation can be obtained only by a chromosome evaluation (karyo-typing). For this, dividing cells are required. The usual source is peripheral blood lymphocytes. A heparinised blood sample should be sent to an appropriate laboratory as soon as it has been collected; a sample from the male co-twin can improve the accuracy of the test.

As the heifer approaches puberty there may be evidence of an enlarged clitoris and increased tufts of hair at the ventral commissure of the vulva. Rectal palpation will reveal the absence of normal structures of the genital tract anterior to the cervix. There will be no normal ovaries and thus no cyclical activity (see section 7.6).

3.6 INITIATION OF PARTURITION

The fetal calf is responsible for the initiation of calving. It triggers a complex cascade of endocrine changes:

(1) During pregnancy the dominant hormone is progesterone, produced by the CL and feto-placental unit (see section 2.10).
(2) Progesterone suppresses cyclical activity, stimulates the changes in the uterus that enable the embryo/fetus to develop, and suppresses myometrial activity which might expel the calf.
(3) As the calf reaches maturity the fetal hypothalamus is stimulated by, or becomes capable of responding to, stimuli which induce the release of adrenocorticotrophic hormone (ACTH) from the fetal pituitary and subsequently corticoids from the fetal adrenal.
(4) The rise in corticosteroids activates the enzyme 17α – hydroxylase which stimulates the conversion of placentally-derived progesterone into oestrogens.
(5) The increase in oestrogens stimulates the synthesis and release of $PGF_2\alpha$ from the placentomes.
(6) Oestrogens also stimulate the synthesis of contractile protein in the myometrium, increase the number of myometrial oxytocin and $PGF_2\alpha$ receptors, increase the number of gap-junctions between smooth muscle fibres and induce softening and ripening of the cervix. Progesterone has the opposite effect.
(7) $PGF_2\alpha$ causes lysis of the CL of pregnancy, induces cervical ripening and causes uterine contractions.
(8) Uterine contractions force the fetus and surrounding fetal membranes against the cervix and anterior vagina, thus stimulating sensory receptors and as a consequence the reflex release of oxytocin (Ferguson's reflex).
(9) Oxytocin stimulates the oestrogen-primed myometrium to contract causing further cervical dilation and expulsion of the fetus.

3.7 SIGNS OF IMPENDING CALVING

These are largely dependent upon hormonal changes; there is considerable variation between individual animals in the extent of the changes and their timing.

- Increased udder development and the presence of colostrum.
- Oedema of the udder and ventral abdominal wall.
- Relaxation of pelvic ligaments, especially sacrosciatic and sacro-iliac.
- Sinking of the sacrosciatic area with apparent elevation of base of tail.
- Relaxation of the perineum and vulva.
- Liquifaction of mucous cervical seal with resultant cloudy mucoid vulval discharge.
- Slight decrease in body temperature.

3.8 FIRST STAGE OF PARTURITION
(Average duration of 6 h; range 1–24 h)

This is difficult to determine in some cows, especially those that have had many calves. It starts with the occurrence of regular, coordinated uterine contractions that increase in frequency and amplitude as the stage progresses. The effects of these are to:

- cause pain and discomfort which result in behaviour changes such as restlessness, inappetence, desire for isolation and solitude, tail twitching, and elevated pulse rate;
- stimulate the calf to alter its disposition within the uterus so that it is capable of passing through the birth canal (see Fig. 9.1);
- dilate the cervix; the external os precedes the internal os;
- push the fetus and its surrounding fetal fluid and fetal membranes towards the cervix and pelvic canal.

3.9 SECOND STAGE OF PARTURITION
(Average duration of 70 min; range 30 min–4 h)

This commences when there is fairly regular and forceful straining, which is stimulated when the fetus and/or fetal membranes enter the pelvic canal. An early consequence is the rupture of the allantochorion with the escape of watery allantoic fluid ('water-bag').

During this stage, the calf is gradually expelled due to straining and also to myometrial contractions. The greatest expulsive effort occurs with the passage of the occiput through the vulva and the thorax through the pelvic canal and vulva.

3.10 THIRD STAGE OF PARTURITION
(Average duration of 6 h)

Uterine contractions continue for several days after the birth of the calf, becoming progressively less frequent and less forceful. These assist in the normal detachment of the placenta which occurs as a result of:

- Ripening and maturation of the placenta due to the endocrine cascade described in section 3.6. Such changes include: flattening of the maternal crypt epithelium; change in the molecular structure of placentome collagen; migration and increased activity of leucocytes; reduction in the number of binucleate cells in the trophectoderm; hyalinisation of placentome blood vessel walls; change in composition of 'glue line' proteins between maternal/fetal epithelium; alloreactivity.
- Rupture of the umbilicus with rapid exsanguination of the fetal side of the placenta with shrinkage of the fetal placental villi.

- Distortion of the caruncle by the myometrial contractions, causing detachment of the cotyledon by separation of the villi from the associated crypts.
- Gravitational pull on the protruding placental mass.
- Persistence of uterine contractions expelling the placental mass.

3.11   CALVING ENVIRONMENT

For successful calving, with the birth of a live calf and the survival of a healthy dam, a good calving environment is necessary. It should also be convenient should problems occur so that early and effective intervention can be made. Calving outside in a well-grassed and well-drained field has much to commend; however, good observation can sometimes prove difficult. When calving indoors the following conditions are necessary:

- The cow should be separated from the rest of the herd at the onset of the first stage (see section 3.7) or earlier.
- A clean, warm, well-ventilated, well-bedded box with adequate lighting and sufficient size to enable obstetrical procedures to be performed (5 m × 4 m).
- A method of restraining the cow by the head (some cows will resent this; thus other methods must be used).
- The ability to observe the cow without causing disturbance.
- Adequate supply of fresh drinking water.
- Absence of protruding objects which might injure the cow, handler or veterinary surgeon.

3.12   PREMATURE INDUCTION OF CALVING

It is possible to induce calving prematurely by administering exogenous hormones, which mimic some of the endocrine changes outlined in section 3.6.

Hormones used in induction

- Adrenocorticotrophic hormone (ACTH), this is not practicable and is too expensive.
- Water-soluble, short-acting corticosteroids, e.g. betamethasone and dexamethasone sodium phosphate, dose of 20–30 mg per cow.
- Medium-acting corticosteroids, e.g. betamethasone and dexamethasone phenyl proprionate with dexathesone sodium phosphate.
- Long-acting corticosteroids, e.g. dexamethasone trimethylacetate, triamcinolone acetonide and flumethasone suspension.
- Prostaglandin $F_2\alpha$ or analogues, e.g. cloprostenol, dinoprost, fenpros-

talene, luprostiol (see section 1.13 for dose rates), or prostaglandin E_2 – not available commercially.

- Combinations of long-acting corticosteroid esters and prostaglandin $F_2\alpha$ and analogues.

Indications for induction

- To reduce the possibility of dystocia due to feto-maternal disproportion associated with prolonged gestation, maternal immaturity, or the conformation of the calf.
- To tighten a seasonal calving pattern by advancing the time of parturition, particularly in order to meet the availability of good pasture growth for milk production.
- To advance the time of calving in a cow suffering from disease or injury so that she can be sent for emergency slaughter.

Requirements

- Known date of natural service or AI or *accurate* estimate.
- At least 260 days' gestation for the birth of viable calves.
- Full discussion between veterinary surgeon and farmer so that the possible consequences of premature induction are known.
- Adequate calving accommodation if groups of animals are induced at the same time.
- Good standard of calf rearing with the availability of skilled husbandmen capable of rearing premature calves.

Procedures

- If corticosteroids are used, cows or heifers should be examined to eliminate the presence of infectious disease. Prophylactic broad-spectrum antibiotics may be used.
- Short-acting corticosteroids will induce calving 2–5 days after injection on or after day 260 of gestation.
- Medium-acting corticosteroids are effective from about day 240 of gestation; the time interval from injection is variable (5–12 days).
- Long-acting corticosteroids are effective at less than 240 days of gestation; the time interval is variable (11–18 days). This is best combined with the administration of $PGF_2\alpha$ or analogue 11 days later which will normally result in calving within 48 h.
- A single dose of prostaglandin $F_2\alpha$ or analogue will induce calving after 255 days of gestation within 2–3 days of injection.

Problems

- Sufficient softening and relaxation of the vulva, perineum and pelvic ligaments does not always occur following the use of prostaglandins. Better results have been obtained with corticosteroids.

- Placental retention is common – the possibility is increased the earlier parturition is induced.
- Uterine involution (see section 5.5) may be delayed and there may be a greater tendency for cows to develop endometritis. There does not appear to be any adverse effect upon subsequent fertility.
- Although there is some evidence for a reduced level of immunoglobulins in colostrum of cows induced with corticosteroids, this does not appear to increase the calves' susceptibility to disease or reduce their viability, provided that they are not very premature.

3.13   DELAYING CALVING

It is possible to delay parturition temporarily so that it does not occur at inconvenient times, especially at night in the absence of adequate super-vision, or perhaps in order to allow adequate relaxation of the vagina, vulva and perineum to occur in heifers. A β_2 agonist, clenbuterol hydrochloride, stimulates the β receptors in the myometrium causing relaxation of smooth muscle and abolishing uterine contractions.

- To postpone parturition: inject 0.3 mg clenbuterol hydrochloride (10 ml) intramuscularly followed by a second injection of 0.21 mg (7 ml) 4 h later; this will inhibit parturition for 8 h after the second injection.
- To improve relaxation: follow a similar regimen with an interval of at least 4 h between successive doses.
- If the cervix is fully dilated and the second stage has commenced (see section 3.9) clenbuterol hydrochloride should not be used.

4   Care of the New-born Calf

4.1   INTRODUCTION

In dealing with a dystocia, or following normal calving, attention must also be paid to the calf and its well-being. Details of normal birth weights are given in Table 3.1.

4.2   ADAPTATION TO THE ENVIRONMENT

During late pregnancy and during the process of parturition the calf undergoes maturational changes that enable it to survive in its new, free-living environment. Many of these are induced by the endocrine changes that initiate the act of parturition (see section 3.6), in particular the rise in the levels of corticosteroids, oestrogens and prostaglandins. Examples of these changes are: development of pulmonary surfactant to allow normal respiration; changes in the haemoglobin composition; ability of the calf to control glucose haemostasis; closure of the foramen ovale and ductus arteriosus.

4.3   PROCEDURES FOLLOWING THE BIRTH OF THE CALF

The following action is necessary:

- Check whether the calf is alive by palpating its heart or carotid pulse, assessing reflexes.
- Clear mucus from external nares and buccal cavity.
- Place calf with head downwards so that fluids can drain from the upper respiratory tract (most of the fluid probably arises from the abomasum).
- Ensure that spontaneous respiration is present and that the airways are clear.
- Check the umbilicus for evidence of haemorrhage from vessels. If severe, clamp and ligate.

- Check for obvious congenital abnormalities (see section 8.11).
- Ensure that the cow will accept the calf so that maternal bonding is established and that she will not attack and injure the calf.
- Check the cow's udder for presence of colostrum.

4.4 PROBLEMS FOLLOWING BIRTH

- Absence of heart beat and pulse. Perform external cardiac massage.
- Obstructed respiratory tract. Use sucker to aspirate fluid from buccal cavity and upper respiratory tract, endotracheal intubation and a source of oxygen. Stimulate cough or sneeze reflex.
- Failure of spontaneous respiration. Perform artificial respiration by compressing the chest, or following endotracheal intubation. Oxygen with a face mask can also be beneficial. Briskly rub the limbs, chest and body surface with straw or a cloth.

    Respiratory stimulants can be used: doxapram hydrochloride by intravenous, intramuscular, subcutaneous or sublingual route at a dose of 40–100 mg (2–5 ml). A mixture of crotethamide and cropropamide as a syrup placed on or under the tongue.
- Respiratory and metabolic acidosis. Calves will have a transient acidosis following a normal calving. Obstetrical manipulations including traction and a caesarean operation will prolong it for several hours. Intravenous sodium bicarbonate can be used to reverse acidosis and prevent long lasting damage, at a dose rate of 5–7 m Eq/kg body weight.
- Failure to accept the calf. Licking of the calf can be stimulated by smearing amniotic fluid around the cow's muzzle and placing the calf near the head. A vicious cow is best sedated.
- Absence of colostrum or failure of let-down. Use bulked, stored colostrum or induce let-down with oxytocin followed by hand milking. Ensure that the calf receives at least 2.5 l of colostrum in the first 6 h of life.
- Calving injuries. Excessive traction badly applied can result in epiphyseal separation, rib or limb bone fracture and femoral nerve paralysis, especially in breeds such as Charolais and Simmental. A substantial number of calf mortalities following dystocia are due to such injuries.

4.5 WEAKLY CALVES

These usually occur as a result of dystocia, perhaps due to some degree of cerebral anoxia, or possibly genetic factors and certain infectious agents. They require much attention to ensure that they are able to suck; if not, hand-rearing with a bottle may be required. If a substantial number of dead or weakly calves are born following normal calving, the presence of a fetopathic infection should be investigated (see sections 8.6 and 8.7). In their absence the presence of trace element deficiencies such as iodine or selenium should be considered.

5 The Post-partum Period (Puerperium)

5.1 INTRODUCTION

The period after calving when the genital tract is returning to its normal non-pregnant state is described as the *puerperium*. In order to obtain optimum fertility, with the cow producing a live calf every 12 months, it is important that this phase of reproductive life is normal in order to ensure that the cow conceives by 85 days after calving (see sections 7.4 and 7.10).

A number of important changes occur during the puerperium. These are:

- Return of normal cyclical ovarian activity.
- Shrinkage of the uterus to its normal non-pregnant state (involution).
- Regeneration of the endometrium.
- Elimination of bacterial contamination.

5.2 RETURN OF NORMAL CYCLICAL OVARIAN ACTIVITY

During pregnancy the ovary ceases to undergo cyclical activity. After calving there is a period of 3–4 weeks in dairy cows (slightly longer in beef suckler cows) before there is the first ovulation, invariably in the ovary opposite the previously gravid uterine horn. The first ovulation frequently occurs with the absence of behavioural signs of oestrus; subsequent ovulations are usually associated with behavioural signs of oestrus.

Evidence of follicular growth can frequently be detected before the first ovulation. In some cows fluid-filled structures > 2.5 cm in diameter can be palpated on the ovaries; these are not true cysts (see sections 7.6 and 7.8) and normally have a short lifespan.

The first cycle after the onset of ovarian activity is often short (15–16 days) because of a reduced luteal phase. Some of these first cycles are associated with the formation of luteinized follicles that behave in a similar fashion to a normal CL. They are *not* cysts because they are < 2.5 cm in diameter; they do not persist or cause aberrant reproductive behaviour (see section 1.14).

5.3   METHODS OF DETERMINING RETURN OF CYCLICAL ACTIVITY

Return of cyclical activity can be assumed to have occurred if a CL can be palpated or identified by ultrasonograph (see Figs 1.16f and g) with certainty on one of the ovaries (the CL of pregnancy *always* regresses just before calving). If a CL cannot be identified then sequential palpations should be performed, or alternatively at least one blood or milk progesterone assay should be carried out 10 days before or after the time of rectal examination.

5.4   FACTORS INFLUENCING RETURN OF CYCLICAL ACTIVITY

- Problems during calving, such as dystocia, metritis, retained placenta or mastitis, will delay the return.
- High milk production may extend the interval to first ovulation.
- Poor nutrition during late pregnancy and after calving can delay return, particularly insufficient energy intake resulting in loss of body condition.
- Breed of cow: beef breeds are slower to return to oestrus than dairy breeds whilst there are also differences between breeds.
- Parity: primipara (first-calf heifers) are acyclic longer than pluripara (more than one calf).
- Season of the year: there is good evidence of the influence of the length of daylight hours.
- Climate: cows return to oestrus earlier in temperate climates than in tropical climates.
- Suckling and frequency of milking: the speed of return is largely inversely proportional to the frequency of milking and intensity of suckling.

5.5   INVOLUTION

Involution, meaning rolling inwards or turning in, is the shrinkage of the uterus to its normal, non-pregnant state. As the uterus shrinks, it becomes more curved or coiled and returns to the pelvic cavity. The cervix, and to a lesser extent the vagina, also undergoes involution.

Initially the process of involution is rapid but the rate gradually declines; it is probably complete by 42 days after calving, although if this is assessed clinically by rectal palpation then changes after 25–30 days are imperceptible (see Fig. 5.1). The cervix also reduces in length and diameter (width) with relatively little change occurring after 25–30 days.

Uterine involution is an active process in which there is extensive loss of collagen and a reduction in the size, and probably the number, of myofibrils in the myometrium. Prostaglandin $F_{2\alpha}$ is produced by the post-partum

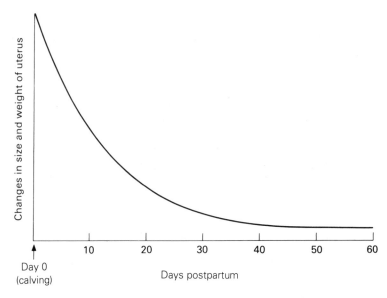

Fig. 5.1 Diagram to show rate of involution of uterus postpartum.

uterus, reaching maximum values 3–4 days after calving and persisting for about 2–3 weeks; it is likely that this hormone is involved in the process of uterine involution, although its specific role is unknown.

Factors influencing rate of involution

- Parity: involution is likely to be more rapid in primipara than pluripara.
- Season of the year: involution is probably quicker in spring- and summer-calving cows.
- Suckling: possibly hastens involution.
- Climate.
- Parturient and periparturient problems, such as dystocia, placenta retention or infection.
- Speed of return to cyclical activity (see section 5.2).
- The administration of exogenous hormones has no influence on uterine involution.

5.6 REGENERATION OF THE ENDOMETRIUM

The cow does not have a true deciduate placenta. However, after calving and placental dehiscence there is necrosis and sloughing of caruncular tissue, followed by regeneration of the endometrium overlying the caruncles.

The changes can be summarised:

- Degenerative changes occur 2 days after calving involving the surface of the caruncle.
- By 5 days after calving the caruncle is covered by a necrotic layer 1–2 mm thick.
- From 5 to 10 days there is sloughing of the necrotic tissue which becomes liquefied and contributes to the lochial discharge or 'second cleansing'.
- From about 15 days there is the beginning of re-epithelisation of the denuded caruncle which is completed by about 25 days.
- The complete restoration of endometrial structure, including the uterine glands, is probably complete by 50–60 days.

Factors delaying regeneration of the endometrium

- Parturient or periparturient problems, such as dystocia, placental retention, trauma or infection.
- Possibly dietary deficiencies.

5.7 BACTERIAL CONTAMINATION

The uterus is sterile during pregnancy; access to the lumen is guarded by the closed cervix and mucous seal. At calving, and immediately post-partum, the cervix is dilated and the vulva and perineum are relaxed, thus allowing the entry of bacteria from faeces and the cow's environment to enter the uterus. Culture from the uterus of most cows after calving will reveal the presence of an extensive, mixed bacterial flora. The main organisms cultured are coliforms, *Actinomyces pyogenes*, streptococci and staphylococci spp., and in some cases anaerobic gram-negative bacteria which are frequently associated with the development of metritis (see sections 11.8 and 11.9).

5.8 ELIMINATION OF BACTERIAL CONTAMINATION

The bacterial flora is a fluctuating one but in most cows the uterus is sterile within 4–5 weeks after calving. Bacteria are eliminated by:

- Physical detachment due to necrosis and sloughing of the surface of the caruncles.
- Physical expulsion associated with the persistent uterine contractions, involution and the lochial discharge.
- Phagocytic activity of the leucocytes that migrate into the uterine lumen.
- Secretory immunoglobulins.

Factors interfering with the elimination of bacteria

- Placental retention.
- Trauma to the genital tract.
- Poor uterine involution.
- Delayed return to oestrus after calving (see sections 11.8 and 11.9).

5.9 FERTILITY POSTPARTUM

Although return to cyclical activity and ovulation has occurred by 3–4 weeks in most dairy cows, optimum fertility as measured by pregnancy rate (see section 7.11) is not reached until 90–100 days after calving. This is because the genital tract environment is either not capable of ensuring that fertilisation can occur, or is not capable of sustaining the developing embryo. However, the improvement in fertility after 50 days postpartum is only relatively small (see Fig. 5.2).

There is no evidence that early breeding after calving will have any cumulative or long-term detrimental effect upon fertility.

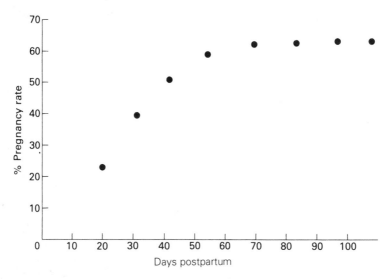

Fig. 5.2. Pregnancy rates relative to time after calving.

6 Lactation

6.1 NORMAL MAMMARY DEVELOPMENT

Before the onset of puberty, the mammary gland grows at the same rate as other body organs. After puberty, because of the secretion of oestrogens (at oestrus) and progesterone (during the luteal phase of the oestrous cycle), together with prolactin and somatotrophin secreted by the anterior pituitary, there is lengthening and branching of the prepubertal juvenile duct system. In addition, there is some alveolar development. During the first four months of pregnancy, when oestrogens are the dominant hormones, there is further expansion of the duct system. During the latter part of gestation, progesterone becomes the dominant reproductive steroid hormone, stimulating the formation of the lobules of the alveolar tissue (site of milk secretion); this increases until term. Other hormones, such as ACTH, thyroid hormones, insulin and adrenal corticosteroids and placental lactogens, also play a role.

The cow's udder is capable of producing milk from about halfway through pregnancy; if abortion occurs after 7 months there is usually sufficient alveolar tissue present to produce modest, though reduced, milk yields.

6.2 LACTOGENESIS

The onset of lactation at the time of calving is due to the endocrine changes that occur around the time of parturition (see section 3.6). To summarise:

- Oestrogens rise towards the end of gestation.
- Progesterone gradually declines and then falls precipitously 24–48 h before calving.
- Corticosteroids rise sharply at calving.
- Prolactin increases 4–6 days before calving.

The key hormone is probably progesterone since, having stimulated alveolar development in late pregnancy, its sudden decline allows prolactin to be released and hence exert its effect. Progesterone also suppresses lactose synthesis in the alveoli; this sugar has an important regulatory role in controlling the secretion of water and the water soluble components of milk. Furthermore, progesterone may also block receptor sites in the udder for cortisol; thus with its demise cortisol can then act upon the mammary gland.

Once lactation has been initiated, prolactin and somatotrophin are the hormones mainly responsible for the maintenance of lactation by controlling the secretory activity of the alveolar epithelium.

6.3   MILK LET-DOWN

Milk secreted by the alveolar tissue accumulates in the collecting ducts, milk sinuses and cisterns (about 80% is stored in the udder in these sites).

Let-down or ejection is largely due to the action of oxytocin and to a lesser extent antidiuretic hormone (ADH). The stimulus for oxytocin release arises from sensory receptors on the udder, teats and genital organs and also as a result of conditioning to sounds and routines associated with suckling or milking.

Oxytocin has a short half-life of less than 2 min in the cow and hence re-stimulation is required.

The milk ejection reflex responsible for milk let-down is readily inhibited by stress, due to the complete or partial blocking of oxytocin secretion from the posterior pituitary by the action of adrenaline.

Induction of let-down

Give 10 iu oxytocin intravenously with repeated injections if necessary. Determine the reason for the inhibition of the milk ejection reflex and try to correct it. In the case of heifers, attempt to establish a conditioning regimen.

6.4   ARTIFICIAL INDUCTION OF LACTATION

This has been tried in dairy cows and heifers for many years by attempting to mimic the endocrine changes that are normally responsible for lactogenesis.

Method A

- A combined injection of 10 mg oestradiol benzoate in oil (2 ml) and 100 mg progesterone in oil (4 ml) is injected subcutaneously on days 0, 3, 6, 9, 12, 15, 18, 21, 24, 27 and 30.
- On days 31 and 32, 20 mg dexamethasone (soluble) is injected intramuscularly.
- From day 10 cows/heifers should be taken through the milking parlour

and milking routine; udders should be massaged and the milking machine applied for short periods.
- Milk production can start before the end of treatment or up to a week after the end.

Method B

- A combined injection at 12-hourly intervals of oestradiol benzoate (0.05 mg kg^{-1}) and progesterone (0.125 mg kg^{-1}) on days 0–7; fourteen injections in total.
- 20 mg of betamethasone or dexamethasone (soluble) by injection on days 18, 19 and 20.
- Udder massage and milking regimen as described in method A.

In both methods cows should have been dry for at least 6 weeks. Milk should be withdrawn from use for 7 days.

Results

- About 20% failure of induction.
- Milk yields are about 70% of predicted yields.
- Subsequent fertility is normal.
- Some cows show evidence of nymphomania during oestrogen therapy.

Indications

- To enable well-bred, high-yielding cows that have failed to conceive to be retained in tightly seasonal calving herds so that they can be bred normally next year.
- To retain high-yielding cows that are infertile or possibly sterile in the herd rather than to purchase expensive replacements.

The procedure is expensive and concern must be expressed at the welfare implications of repeated injections. It will not replace pregnancy and parturition as the method of stimulating lactation.

Recombinant-derived bovine somatotrophin administered parenterally will increase milk yields in dairy cows by up to 25% or more. It exerts an effect by directing nutrients away from body deposition to milk production. Treated cows must be fed adequate concentrate rations and good quality forage. It is not licensed in many parts of the world.

7 Fertility and Infertility in the Cow

7.1 DEFINITIONS

- *Fertility* is the ability of a cow to give birth to a live calf at approximately 12-monthly intervals.
- *Sterility* is the total inability of a cow to become pregnant and to give birth to a live calf.
- *Infertility or subfertility* is reduced fertility, i.e. the cow is ultimately capable of becoming pregnant and giving birth to a live calf but the interval may be much longer than 12 months.

7.2 INFERTILITY AND CULLING

Aside from the current exceptional situation in the UK, where cows are being slaughtered as part of the Government scheme to try to accelerate the elimination of BSE from the national herd, between a quarter and a third of the dairy cows that are culled annually in the UK are culled because of breeding problems. Some of these cows are sterile; the majority, however, are infertile or subfertile but, because of the economic loss associated with poor reproductive performance they are culled rather than given sufficient time to become pregnant. Some cows are culled because problems may be anticipated, e.g. perhaps the cow suffered from trauma at calving or severe post-partum infection (see sections 11.3, 11.6 and 11.8).

7.3 EXPECTATIONS FOR FERTILITY – THE INDIVIDUAL COW

In any normal population of cows it is unlikely that the average calving rate to each insemination will be much greater than 55% (i.e. if a hundred cows are inseminated once then only fifty-five will subsequently give birth to a calf). The reasons for the 45% that fail to calve are:

- About 10–15% of ovulated oocytes are not fertilised.

- About 15–20% of fertilised oocytes or early embryos die before day 13 of the oestrous cycle.
- About 10% of late embryos die between days 14 and 42.
- About 5% of fetal death occurs after 42 days.

When fertilisation fails to occur, or where early embryonic death occurs, cows will return to oestrus at the normal interval of 18–24 days (25–35%) and, if observed, should be re-inseminated. The same probabilities are likely following the second and subsequent inseminations. Thus in any herd with normal fertility at least 6% of the cows will require more than three inseminations although they are completely normal from a reproductive point of view.

7.4   THE REASONS FOR A 12-MONTH INTERVAL BETWEEN CALVINGS

A 12-month (365-day) interval between successive calvings is the optimum, except for cows in their first lactation or for high-yielding individuals (>8000kg per lactation), when an interval of 13 months or longer is more suitable. Reasons for a 12-month interval are:

- There is a greater yield from 305-day lactation.
- Calving occurs at the same time each year so as to utilise the available feed effectively.
- It enables calves to be reared in groups of similar age and body weight.

7.5   FACTORS RESPONSIBLE FOR INFERTILITY

A request to examine an infertile cow usually arises because she does not appear to fit the agreed targets for the herd – in particular, she is unlikely to produce a calf approximately 12 months after she has given birth to the previous one. Alternatively, she may be identified because she is showing some abnormal reproductive behaviour.

It is proposed to deal with the individual cow as she would appear to the herdsman responsible for managing her breeding programme. Before reading the section it may be worth consulting Chapters 1 and 5.

7.6   NO SIGNS OF OESTRUS – APPROACH AND CLINICAL EXAMINATION

Once puberty has occurred at 7–18 months of age (see section 1.1), the heifer should have cyclical ovarian activity. In the absence of reproductive disorders or severe intercurrent disease the only two occasions when this does not occur are during pregnancy and for a short time after calving (see section 5.2). In all animals with no signs of oestrus *pregnancy must always be eliminated as a cause before therapy is implemented* (see section 2.11).

General bodily condition (condition score) and general health should be assessed and current milk yield determined. A thorough palpation of the ovaries and tubular genital tract should be performed, together with transrectal ultrasound imaging, if the equipment is available; a repeat examination may be necessary.

Heifers

- *No ovarian tissue palpable*: ovarian agenesis which is very rare; animal should be culled.
- *Small, spindle-shaped ovaries with normal but infantile tubular genital tract*: ovarian hypoplasia, which is rare, or delayed puberty. Estimate body weight and compare with heifers of similar age and size. If delayed puberty, further growth should alleviate the problem.
- *Small, spindle-shaped structures where ovaries should be sited normally and absence of normal tubular genitalia* represents a freemartin. Enquire if it was purchased from a market or dealer. Examine external genitalia, especially the clitoris which may be larger or more prominent than normal. Single-born freemartins can occur (see section 3.5). Confirm by karyotyping. There is no treatment.

Heifers and cows

Check bodily condition and perform rectal palpation of the whole reproductive system. Eliminate pregnancy as a cause. Transrectal ultrasound imaging of the ovaries might be useful, if the equipment is available.

- *Small, smooth and flattened ovaries with normal tubular genitalia*: likely to be acyclic (true anoestrus). Confirmation may require a second rectal examination or a milk/blood progesterone assay 10 days later; an elevated progesterone value will indicate the presence of cyclical activity.

  Increase energy intake if appetite permits; in high-yielding cows it may be necessary to wait until yield declines. Severe trace element deficiencies, such as copper or cobalt, and chronic parasitism might be responsible in heifers.

  Stimulate ovarian activity by inserting a PRID (see section 1.12) which is withdrawn after 12 days with oestrus occurring within 3–4 days; 600 iu eCG on the day of removal might be beneficial, or, a CIDR (see section 1.12) for 7 days followed by 1mg oestradiol benzoate 3 days after removal, or, GnRH analogue with oestrus 1–3 weeks later.

- *Usually one, but occasionally both, ovaries will be large (4–5 cm in length) and contain a fluid-filled structure > 2.5 cm in diameter*: this is a cyst which arises as a result of failure of ovulation of a follicle, which does not regress and becomes atretic, but continues to grow and persists. They are frequently thick-walled (Fig. 7.1a, b) and can be identified using transrectal ultrasonography as being > 3 mm (see Fig. 1.16j).

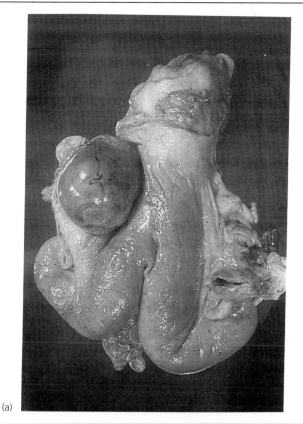

(a)

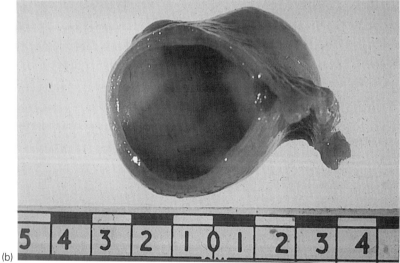

(b)

Fig. 7.1. (a) Genital tract of cow with pathologically-enlarged right ovary due to the presence of a luteal cyst. (b) Section of ovary with a luteal cyst; note the diameter of the cyst is about 4 cm with a wall of almost 5 mm thickness due to the presence of luteal tissue. (Courtesy of Dr T.J. Parkinson.)

Confirmation of the structure as a luteal or luteinised cyst can be made following a milk or blood progesterone assay which will show high progesterone concentrations.

Treat with prostaglandin $F_2\alpha$ or analogue which will cause regression and oestrus in 2–3 days; serve at observed oestrus. Cysts will often recur.

Sometimes cysts are present but milk or blood progesterone assays show low or basal levels; these are follicular cysts with a wall < 3mm when imaged ultrasonographically (see Fig. 1.16i) and do not respond to prostaglandin therapy. Treatment with GnRH analogue or human chorionic gonadotrophin (hCG) causes luteinisation; 10 days later $PGF_2\alpha$ or analogue can be used to cause regression of this structure or insert a PRID for 12 days.

- *CL on one or both ovaries*: eliminate the presence of pregnancy as the cause. The most likely cause is non-detection of oestrus (see section 1.8). However, it may be due to the cow failing to show oestrous behaviour (sub-oestrus or silent heat) or very rarely it is a persistent CL.

  Non-detection of oestrus is generally a herd management problem. If it is an isolated animal, treat with prostaglandin $F_2\alpha$, or analogue, serve at observed oestrus, usually 3–5 days later, or if no observed oestrus, repeat prostaglandin $F_2\alpha$ after 11 days followed by fixed-time AI (see sections 1.11–1.13). PRIDs may be used (see section 1.12), preferably in association with $PGF_2\alpha$ or analogue administered approximately 24 hours before removal. If it is a herd problem then ensure that true signs of oestrus are known and that a regular routine is used, or use oestrus detection aids (see sections 1.8 and 1.9).

  Apart from the first, and less frequently the second, ovulation it is rare for it not to be preceded by behavioural signs of oestrus. Frequently sub-oestrus or silent oestrus is used to excuse poor detection; however, some cows can be missed because of the short duration or weak expression of behavioural signs. Treat with prostaglandin $F_2\alpha$ or analogue or PRID, as for non-detected oestrus; in addition, an oestrus-detection aid, such as a KaMaR, can be used at the same time (see section 1.9).

  A persistent CL is very rare in the absence of uterine lesions since it must occur as a result of the failure of release of endogenous prostaglandin (see section 1.7). Palpate uterine horns for disparity in size and thickened, oedematous walls; distinguish from pregnancy (see section 2.11). The most likely reason for the persistent CL will be postpartum uterine infection, especially pyometra (see Fig. 7.2) (see section 11.10). Vaginal examination may reveal a purulent discharge. Treat with prostaglandin $F_2\alpha$ or analogue, request that the cow is carefully observed for the presence of a vulval discharge, and re-examine her about 10 days later.

- *Ovaries are small but round and active; there is good to moderate uterine tone*: the cow or heifer may be coming into oestrus, is in oestrus or is in early metoestrus. Look for signs of the animal being ridden and

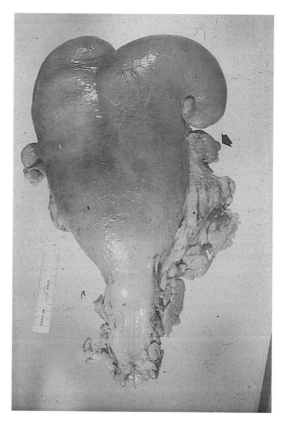

Fig. 7.2 Genital tract of cow with pyometra and persistent CL in the right ovary (arrow). Note fibrin tags on the serosal surface of the uterine horns.

evidence of mucus on the tail or perineum; part the labiae of the vulva and look for the presence of oestral mucus or metoestral bleeding (see section 1.8).

A positive diagnosis can frequently be difficult following a single examination, hence a re-examination or milk/blood progesterone assay in 10 days should confirm the presence of a CL and indicate normal cyclical activity.

7.7   REGULAR RETURN TO OESTRUS

The cow or heifer returns to oestrus regularly at the normal interval (18–24 days) after each insemination. This can be due to *failure of fertilisation or early embryonic death* (before day 14) when the maternal recognition of pregnancy occurs (see section 2.9).

Failure of fertilisation

It is necessary to eliminate male causes before proceeding to investigate the cow or heifer; these are as follows:

- *Infertile bull.* Examine breeding records or other females served by the bull for pregnancy. If a considerable number – or all – are not pregnant then the bull must be examined in detail (see Chapter 15).
- *DIY-AI.* Check that the semen storage, handling and insemination technique is correct. If only an isolated cow or heifer returns to oestrus, examine to see if she is difficult to inseminate (see section 14.4).
- *AI from an approved centre.* It should be possible to eliminate the bull and AI techniques as causes of the problem.

Once male factors have been excluded the following approach should be followed in cows and heifers: on rectal palpation the ovaries are likely to be found to be normal and showing evidence of cyclical activity. Careful palpation of the tubular genital tract may indicate segmental aplasia; see if there is accumulation of fluid at any part of the tract. Assess cervical patency with a catheter.

In most cows there will be no abnormalities detectable following rectal palpation, ultrasonography and vaginal exploration. Fertilisation failure may be due to:

- *Acquired lesions,* such as adhesions of the ovary and bursa, uterine tubes and horns, or distention and enlargement of the uterine tubes (Figs. 7.3, 7.4 and 7.5). These lesions either completely occlude the tubular genital tract, and hence prevent spermatozoa and oocyte from

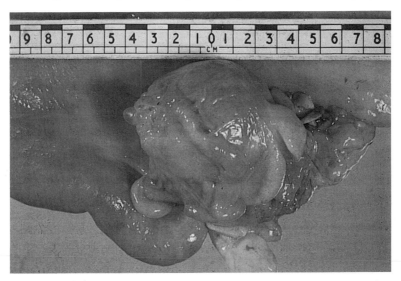

Fig. 7.3. Ovary of cow showing ovaro-bursal adhesions with the ovarian bursa surrounding the ovary and distended uterine tube. (Courtesy of Dr T.J. Parkinson.)

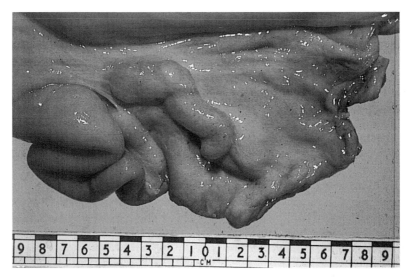

Fig. 7.4 Ovaro-bursal adhesions and distended uterine tube due to hydro- or pyosalpinx. (Courtesy of Dr T.J. Parkinson.)

meeting, or more frequently interfere with normal function, particularly oocyte or sperm transport. Confirmation of occlusion can be obtained by using the phenolsulphonphthalein (PSP) dye test. There is no treatment.

- *Anovulation* is where the mature Graafian follicle fails to ovulate (see section 1.5); it subsequently regresses and becomes atretic. Follicular growth with regression and atresia occurs continuously throughout the oestrous cycle (see section 1.5). However, normally after oestrus at least one mature follicle ovulates to liberate the oocyte and forms a CL.

  Anovulation is most likely to occur in the immediate postpartum period. It can also be followed by the formation of luteinised follicles (see section 5.2) or the follicle can grow and become cystic (see sections 7.6 and 7.8).

  Accurate diagnosis can only be made by sequential rectal palpation or, more accurately, with transrectal ultrasonography, when the follicle will be noted to persist longer than normal in the absence of a developing CL which could also be confirmed using milk or plasma progesterone assays.

  Treat with GnRH analogue or hCG if it occurs repeatedly.

- *Delayed ovulation* implies that ovulation occurs later than the normal 12–15 h after the end of oestrus. Although spermatozoa are capable of fertilisation 30–48 h after insemination there is a decline in their capacity by 15–20 h (see section 2.2). Thus if ovulation is delayed the spermatozoa may be incapable of fertilisation; furthermore, the oocyte might have aged and also be incapable of being fertilised.

  An accurate diagnosis is difficult and can only be done by sequential

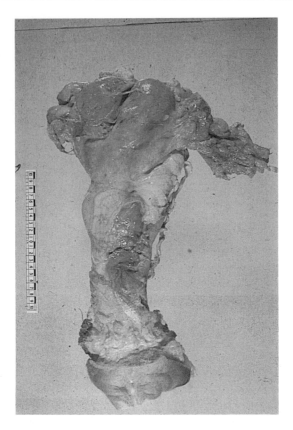

Fig. 7.5 Genital tract of cow with perimetritis. Note extensive adhesions. (Courtesy of Dr T.J. Parkinson.)

rectal palpation or ultrasonography; such techniques might interfere with the timing of ovulation. Its occurrence is based largely on anecdotal evidence. Treat with GnRH analogue or hCG at the time of insemination.
- *An abnormal uterine environment* may be due to an endocrine asynchrony imbalance or chronic infection.

Sperm and oocyte transport is influenced by the hormonal status of the cow. Asynchrony or imbalance is almost impossible to diagnose and cannot be corrected.

Uterine infection (see sections 5.7 and 11.9) may interfere with sperm transport but is more likely to cause death of the spermatozoa. It is unlikely to persist after one or two oestrous periods because of the therapeutic effect of oestrus and is unlikely to be present in the absence of clinical signs. It might occur in association with a vaginitis due to a pneumovagina caused by calving injuries to the vulva (see section 11.2) or urovagina where urine pools in the anterior vagina. Pneumovagina can be corrected surgically (see section 11.2). Urovagina cannot be treated.

Early embryonic death

When the embryo dies before day 14 of the oestrous cycle then the lifespan of the CL is not prolonged and the cow returns to oestrus at a normal interval (see section 2.9). It is not possible to know if early embryonic death is occurring or if there is a failure of fertilisation. As described in section 7.3, a certain level of early embryonic death is normal; there is no explanation for the phenomenon.

Possible reasons for early embryonic death are as follows:

- *Developmental abnormalities due to genetic incompatability* may be responsible so that abnormal embryos develop. It is difficult to prove, however, in a cow that regularly returns to oestrus; the use of a different sire, perhaps from a different breed, may be worthwhile.
- *Stress*: extremes of ambient temperature, transportation, sudden environmental changes or alterations in diet can act as stressors, although their effects are difficult to quantify. Other undetected factors are also likely to be involved.
- *Infection resulting in Pyrexia.*
- *Fatty liver disease* occurs in cows that are over-fat at the time of calving but are fed insufficient energy after calving in early lactation.
- *Nutritional deficiencies and excesses* probably exert an effect upon embryonic survival by their influence upon the uterine environment. Sudden changes in diet during the critical early embryonic phase should be avoided.

  Probably the most important single dietary factor is energy, a factor that can be particularly important in high-yielding cows, because of their inability to consume enough to satisfy the requirements for lactation. There is weight loss after calving which is not usually reversed much before 60 days postpartum; estimation of body condition or weighing is important. Growing animals, especially first-calvers, are particularly susceptible.

  Both protein deficiency and excess can be responsible for early embryonic death; in the case of the latter, excess degradable protein, particularly in association with inadequate energy, can result in increased urea and ammonia production in the rumen. Should elevated levels in the blood result in these substances reaching the uterine lumen, reduced fertility due to their adverse effect upon spermatozoa, oocytes or embryos may occur. Trace element and vitamin deficiencies if home-produced forage and concentrates form a large proportion of the diet can also cause early embryonic death. Dairy cows fed purchased concentrate feeds are unlikely to suffer from such deficiencies.

  Nutritional problems usually affect the whole herd or a major group within the herd.

- *Infection and endocrine imbalance* probably create an adverse environment within the uterus that prevents the normal development of the embryo. This is probably not a very common cause of early embryonic death.

- *Luteal deficiency* may result in embryonic death although it is difficult to prove. A progesterone-dominated uterus is necessary for the survival of the embryo and hence the maintenance of pregnancy. LH is luteotrophic in the cow. hCG can be injected about day 14 of the cycle when the CL would be starting to regress if the cow were not pregnant. This treatment is very empirical. More recently, GnRH analogues have been used, with some success, on days 11–13 after insemination, to improve pregnancy rates (see section 7.10 'Pregnancy rate'). Such treatment around the time of the maternal recognition of pregnancy (see section 2.9) either stimulates accessory CL formation or more likely delays luteolysis for a sufficient length of time to allow the embryo to survive and signal its presence.

7.8 SHORT INTEROESTROUS INTERVAL

The normal interoestrous interval is 18–24 days. Intervals less than 18 days are abnormal except for the first cycle after calving (see section 5.1). The reasons for short intervals are:

- *Follicular cysts* which occur as a result of anovulation (see section 7.7). One or both ovaries will be large (4–5 cm in diameter) and contain one or more fluid-filled structures > 2.5 cm in diameter; they are usually thin-walled and fluctuate when palpated (Fig 7.6a and b).

  The cow will have a history of nymphomania, apparently returning to oestrus every few days, although the main behavioural sign will be the excessive and indiscriminate mounting and riding of other cows. There may be excessive vulval mucus discharge.

  Treatment is with GnRH or hCG to cause luteinisation with subsequent cessation of the nymphomaniacal behaviour. This luteinised structure will often regress spontaneously after 2–3 weeks. A PRID will readily stop behavioural problems with regression of the cyst and the cow will return to oestrus with ovulation 3–5 days after its withdrawal.

  Cysts should not be intentionally ruptured by squeezing per rectum.

- *Incorrect identification and recording of oestrus* can result in short intervals of less than 18 days; the interval either before or after will invariably be extended (25–35 days) which when both are summed will be about 42 days. In most herds there will be a few animals with such records; however, when large numbers of short intervals are recorded it points to a need to improve oestrus detection (see sections 7.6 and 7.10). In order to confirm inaccurate detection of oestrus, milk samples should be collected at the time of insemination for progesterone assays. (see section 2.11); these will have high concentration rather than the normal low at or just after oestrus.

7.9 PROLONGED INTEROESTROUS INTERVAL

Prolonged interoestrous intervals, i.e. > 24 days, are due to the following:

- *Failure to detect oestrus*. In these cases the interval will be a multiple of 18–24 days, that is 36–48 days where one oestrus is missed or perhaps 54–72 days if two are missed. The genital tract and ovaries will be normal on clinical examination. If only a small number of animals are involved then oestrus can be induced with prostaglandin $F_2\alpha$ or analogues (if a CL is present) or with a PRID (see section 1.12). If large numbers are involved then attention must be paid to improving oestrus detection (see sections 1.8, 1.9 and 7.6).
- *Incorrect identification of oestrus*. The cow has been in oestrus but not observed, and then has been incorrectly identified at some stage in the subsequent dioestrus. Intervals can vary between 25 and 35 days or 49 and 53 days (see section 7.8). Individual cows can be treated with prostglandin $F_2\alpha$ or analogues (if a CL is present) or with PRIDs. If large numbers are involved, oestrus detection must be improved (see sections 1.9 and 7.10).
- *Late embryonic or early fetal death*. About 10% of late embryos die between 14 and 42 days; a smaller percentage of early fetal death occurs after this stage (see section 7.3). In all cases the lifespan of the CL is extended, hence the prolonged interval between successive heats. The causes are the same as those described as being responsible for early embryonic death (see section 7.7) and in most cases no specific cause can be found.

    If large numbers of animals in a herd are involved and if natural service is used and cows have a history of a mucopurulent vulval discharge or abortions, then *Campylobacter fetus venerealis* or *Tritrichomonas fetus* infection should be suspected and further investigations performed to confirm its absence or presence (see section 8.6).

7.10 EVALUATING HERD FERTILITY

Before attempting to evaluate the fertility of the whole herd, it is necessary to have accurate records of the reproductive data of all cows. Sometimes these will be readily available, in other cases it will be necessary to glean whatever information is available from such sources as AI certificates or milk records. Ideally, the following data should be recorded: identity of the cow, parity, calving date, dates of first and subsequent services, sire identity, and result of pregnancy test.

In sections 7.1 and 7.4 fertility was defined in relation to the ability of a cow to produce a live calf every 12 months and the reasons for this interval were stated. The interval in days from one calving to the next in an individual cow is referred to as the *calving interval*. It is a useful measure of fertility for an individual animal and should be 365 days.

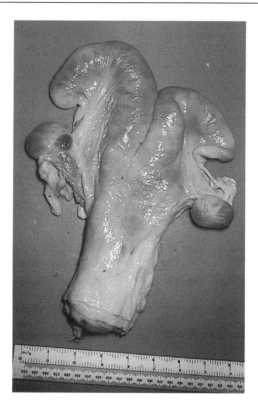

Fig. 7.6. (a) Genital tract of cow with signs of nymphomania with both ovaries enlarged with several follicular cysts.

Having collected whatever data are available, it is now possible to make some simple calculations to obtain a number of different indices which are measurements of the herd's fertility.

- *Calving index* is calculated as the mean calving intervals of all cows in the herd at a specific time calculated retrospectively from their most recent calving at that time. It should be 365 days. The calving index is of limited value because it is an historical measure calculated retrospectively. Thus it does not include cows that currently have not become pregnant or have taken a long time to become pregnant, and furthermore it can flatter the fertility of the herd if large numbers of barren cows are culled. Once a cow has been confirmed pregnant it is possible to calculate a *predicted calving interval* on the assumption that the cow will calve in 280 days time; the *predicted calving index* can be calculated as the mean.
- *Calving-to-conception interval* is the interval in days from calving to the fertile insemination. This is a more immediate measure of fertility, and since the mean length of gestation is fixed at about 280 days then a mean calving-to-conception interval of 85 days will give a calving index of 365 days.

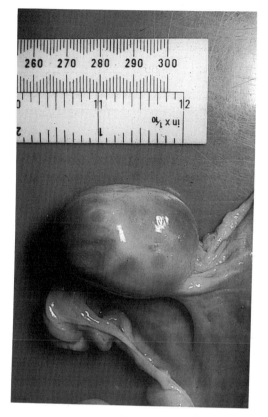

Fig. 7.6. (b) Ovary of nymphomaniacal cow with several thin-walled, follicular cysts.

The calving-to-conception interval will be influenced by how soon cows are served after calving – *calving-to-first-service interval* – and how readily they become pregnant – *pregnancy rate*.

- *Calving-to-first-service interval* is the number of days from calving to the first service postpartum. In order to achieve an 85-day calving-to-conception interval cows should be served from about 45–50 days after calving.

The calving-to-first-service interval will be influenced by:

(1) the time of return to normal cyclical ovarian activity (see sections 5.1 and 7.6);

(2) the detection of cows in oestrus after calving (see sections 1.8 and 7.9);

(3) type of animal – first calvers and high-yielding cows frequently need longer before first service (see section 7.4);

(4) the need to alter or maintain the calving pattern of a herd, e.g. to concentrate the period of calving in a herd.

- *Pregnancy rate* (this used to be referred to as conception rate) can be calculated for first service or all services. It is the number of services that result in a confirmed pregnancy expressed as a percentage of the total number of services. It should be about 60% for first services and 55% for all services.

    The pregnancy rate will be reduced by;

    (1) failure of fertilisation (see section 7.7);
    (2) embryonic or fetal death (see sections 7.7 and 7.9).

- The early and accurate detection of oestrus is important in ensuring optimum fertility. It is possible to make an estimate of the efficiency of both from data collected from herd records. The *oestrus detection rate* is an estimate of the number of oestrous periods detected over a given period expressed as a percentage of the total number that occurred over the same period. This is calculated by counting the number of recorded oestrous periods or services and counting the number of supposedly missed oestrous periods (see section 7.9) over the same period of time. The detection rate should be about 80%, but in many herds it is rarely better than 50% or 60%. Poor oestrus detection can be identified on a farm when large percentages of cows that are not pregnant are presented for routine pregnancy diagnosis at 6–8 weeks.

    Cows are sometimes artificially inseminated when in dioestrus (see section 7.9). A measure of the *accuracy or efficiency of detecting and identifying true oestrus* can be obtained by calculating the inter-oestrus and interservice intervals. The numbers of intervals are summed in the various groups: (a) 2–17 days, (b) 18–24 days, (c) 25–35 days, (d) 36–48 days and (e) > 48 days.

    The *efficiency of oestrus detection* is calculated thus:

$$\frac{b + d}{a + b + c + 2(d + e)} \times 100\%$$

In a good herd a figure of 42 or more will be obtained, in a poor herd it will be 31 or less.

    The figure obtained is only a guide and cannot be considered to be more than an estimate.

    A useful measure of the efficiency of identifying cows in oestrus and having them served is the first service *submission rate*. This is particularly useful in a seasonally calved herd and is defined as the number of cows served within a 21-day period expressed as a percentage of the number of cows at or beyond their earliest service date after calving at the start of the same 21-day period. It should be between 80% and 90%.

- *Culling rate* for those cows that fail to become pregnant is also a useful measure of the overall fertility of a herd. About 95% of cows that calve should ultimately become pregnant again.

7.11   MONITORING AND MAINTAINING GOOD FERTILITY

In a herd that has had poor fertility which has been corrected, or in a herd that has good fertility, it is important to maintain the status. The keys to monitoring and maintaining good fertility are:

- accurate, permanent recording of all relevant data;
- early identification of infertile cows;
- regular, routine visits to examine infertile cows and others.

An efficient scheme can only be implemented with the enthusiasm and cooperation of herdsman, farmer and veterinary surgeon.

Accurate and permanent records

The following data should be recorded:

- Identity of cow; good, clear identification is important.
- Number of calves/lactations.
- Calving date and details of such events as dystocia, retained fetal membranes and uterine infection.
- Dates of observed oestrus before the earliest service date.
- Date of first service and subsequent services (bull identity if possible).
- Confirmation of pregnancy including identification of method used.

These should be recorded in writing immediately they are known and transferred to a book, herd-sheet, individual animal card or computer database. Where data are dispatched to a computer bureau a duplicate should be kept.

From the data listed above it should be possible to calculate the necessary indices that can be used to measure fertility. Rolling means can be obtained and the various indices calculated in relation to the weeks or months of the year. This is particularly useful when they are related to various changes in herd management, such as housing the cows in the autumn, turning them out in the spring, opening a new silage clamp, feeding new concentrate mixtures, or the introduction of a new herdsman or bull.

Cows requiring examination

These should be identified from the data recorded and will include:

- Cows that have suffered from dystocia, retained placenta or metritis: they should be examined 5–6 weeks after calving even if they have not shown any other problems.
- Cows that have an abnormal vulval discharge, such as leucorrhoea (see sections 11.9 and 11.10).
- Cows that have aborted (early investigation will have been undertaken, see sections 8.5 and 8.6).

- Cows that have shown signs of nymphomania (see section 7.8).
- Cows that have not been seen in oestrus by 42 days after calving or have not been served by 63 days after calving (see section 7.6).
- Cows that have been served but have not been seen in oestrus for 42 days, i.e. have missed two consecutive oestrous periods. These cows should be pregnant (see section 2.11) or have not been seen in oestrus (see section 7.6) or are acyclic (see section 7.6).
- Cows that have returned to oestrus at least three times after service (see sections 7.3 and 7.7).
- Cows that have been diagnosed pregnant but have subsequently shown signs of oestrus (see section 2.11).

Frequency of veterinary visits

This will depend upon herd size and the seasonal pattern of calving. Obviously large herds with a very intensive calving season will require at least once-weekly visits which can be reduced in frequency when the majority of the cows are confirmed pregnant.

Recording systems

These have to suit the farm, the number of cows in the herd and the personnel involved in looking after the herd. Avoid complex recording schemes; they should be simple and straightforward.

Computerised recording, particularly computer print-outs, can deter some people. Sophisticated computer programs have the advantage of being able to calculate a large number of indices and frequently to display them graphically. However, the results are only as reliable as the accuracy of the initial data.

8 Problems During Pregnancy

8.1 PRENATAL DEATH

As indicated in section 7.3, not all cows that become pregnant give birth to a live calf at term. Prenatal death can occur at any stage of gestation; therefore the consequences are variable and can involve the early or late embryo, the fetus resulting in abortion, mummification or maceration or the full-term calf that is stillborn.

Early embryonic death
The embryo dies before day 13. It, together with the associated membranes, undergoes autolysis and is resorbed. The cow returns to oestrus at a normal interval and hence it is impossible to differentiate it from fertilisation failure (see section 7.7).

Obviously if the normal interoestrus-interval is greater than the average, and yet still within the normal range (see section 1.3), embryonic death can occur later than 13 days and can still result in a return to oestrus at a normal interval.

Late embryonic death
The embryo dies between days 13 and 42, the fetal fluids are resorbed, and the embryo and its associated membranes undergo autolysis. There may be a slight vulval discharge and the voiding of small quantities of fetal tissue which in most cases will not be observed. The cow returns to oestrus after a prolonged and irregular interval (see section 7.9).

8.2 CAUSES OF EMBRYONIC DEATH

These are listed in sections 7.7 and 7.9 and are:

- Genetic factors.
- Stress.
- Infection resulting in pyrexia.
- Fatty liver disease.

- Nutritional deficiencies and excesses.
- Endocrine deficiencies, asynchrony and imbalance.
- Non-specific infectious agents.
- Specific infectious agents.

Specific infectious agents responsible for embryonic death

- *Tritrichomonas fetus.*
- *Campylobacter fetus venerealis.*
- Bovine viral diarrhoea (BVD) virus.
- Infectious bovine rhinotracheitis (IBR), bovine herpes virus 1 (BHV-1).
- Catarrhal vagino-cervicitis.
- *Chlamydia psittaci.*
- *Haemophilus somnus.*

8.3 FETAL DEATH

Fetal death occurs between day 43 of gestation and term. The consequences are:

- Early fetal death can be followed by expulsion of fetal fluids, autolysis of fetal tissue and membranes which are voided and are sometimes not detected.
- Mummification.
- Abortion.
- Stillbirth.
- Fetal maceration.

8.4 FETAL MUMMIFICATION

After fetal death there is expulsion of fetal fluids, dehydration of fetal tissue and associated membranes, and persistence of the CL of pregnancy so that the products of conception are retained within the uterus.

The condition will be identified when a cow:

- fails to calve at the expected time;
- fails to show udder development and other changes that might be expected towards the last trimester of pregnancy.

On rectal palpation a hard mass will be identified in the uterus with the uterine wall tightly contracted around it; the uterus and contents are readily palpable without the need for retraction. No caruncles or cotyledons will be palpable and there will be no evidence of fremitus in the middle uterine artery (see section 2.11).

The fetal mummy will be expelled following treatment with prostaglandin $F_2\alpha$ or analogue (see section 3.12) within 2–5 days although, because it is dehydrated, assistance may be needed in the form of lubrication and traction per vaginum (Fig. 8.1).

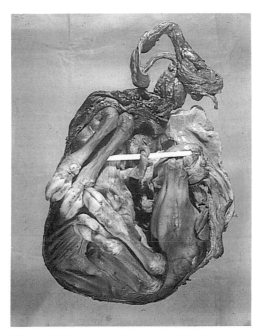

Fig. 8.1 Mummified calf. Note umbilical cord identified by the white marker.

In most cases a specific cause of fetal death with mummification cannot be found. Infectious agents can usually be excluded since they generally cause abortion (see section 8.5).

8.5 ABORTION

Abortion is defined as the expulsion of one or more calves less than 271 days after service or AI; they are either dead or live for less than 24 h.

Frequency
A level of sporadic abortion of 1–2% of pregnant cows is normal; however, if it exceeds 3–5% then a thorough investigation is necessary. Stillbirths and premature calvings must also be taken into consideration.

8.6 ACTION TO BE TAKEN FOLLOWING AN ABORTION

Under the Brucellosis Orders of 1979 (Scotland) and 1981 (England and Wales) *all* births before 271 days constitute an abortion, whether the calf is alive or dead, and under these regulations the following measures must be implemented:

(1) A veterinary inspector or officer (usually the Divisional Veterinary Officer) of the Ministry of Agriculture, Fisheries and Food (MAFF) must be notified.
(2) The cow that is aborting or has aborted must be isolated together with the fetus or calf and placenta.
(3) The fetus or calf and placenta must be retained on the premises.

Readers should check on the current, up-to-date regulations concerning the control of brucellosis.

Irrespective of the statutory requirements under the Brucellosis Orders, good and careful hygiene is necessary to prevent the possibility of lateral spread of an infectious agent, should it be responsible for causing the abortion. If an infectious agent is confirmed, or if there is any suspicion that one might be involved, the following should be implemented:

(1) The placenta and fetal calf should be disposed of by incineration or deep burial.
(2) The contaminated buildings or boxes should be cleaned and disinfected.
(3) Straw, litter or feed that might have become contaminated must be burnt.
(4) Manure or slurry should be disposed of so that there is little chance of the infectious agent being spread.

In some countries an abortion is defined as occurring before 260 days.

Abortions and herd records
If abortion occurs before 152 days there is no need to start a new fertility record. If it occurs after 152 days then a new record commences from the date of the abortion as if the cow had calved normally on that date.

8.7 CAUSES OF ABORTION

Abortion is caused either (a) by infectious agents or (b) by non-infectious agents.

Infectious causes of abortion
A wide range of bacteria, viruses, protozoa and fungi can cause abortion. The frequency with which they occur varies from country to country. In

addition, there will also be changes in the frequency of occurrence due to such factors as: disease eradication schemes, vaccination programmes, changes in husbandry systems, and climate. Identification of specific organisms responsible for abortion can be difficult, with positive results in as few as 6% of calf fetopathies, which is much lower than in other species.

- Spirochaetes of the species *Leptospira interrogans* are a common cause of abortion, stillborn and weakly live calves. A number of serovars have been implicated: *pomona, canicola, icterohaemorrhagiae, grippotyphosa* and *hardjo*; the latter is endemic in the UK and many parts of the world. Abortions, which occur from 4 months to term (most common after 6 months), may follow an acute fever or an afebrile disease sometimes associated with agalactia or 'leptospiral mastitis'. Diagnosis is based upon: identifying leptospires in fetal organs directly or by culture or immunofluorescent techniques; fetal serology. Maternal serology is of little value in identifying individually affected animals but is suitable for herd screening. Treatment and control is by good hygiene, rodent control, segregation of cattle from pigs and possibly sheep, vaccination and streptomycin/dihydrostreptomycin. Leptospirosis is an important zoonosis.
- *Salmonella dublin* is responsible for about 80% of *Salmonella*-induced abortions. It occurs usually sporadically after a bout of severe diarrhoea. The disease often follows access to contaminated pasture or water sources. Abortion occurs most commonly at about 7 months of gestation but it can be variable. Diagnosis is generally based upon isolation of the organism from the fetus, fetal membranes or uterine discharges. Control involves the implementation of good hygiene.
- *Salmonella typhimurium* and other *Salmonellae* are less commonly responsible for abortion than *S. dublin*. Diagnosis and control is similar to that used for *S. dublin*.
- *Bacillus licheniformis* has been identified as a common cause of sporadic abortion in cattle over the last 10 years. Infection occurs as a result of ingestion of water and food often contaminated with silage effluent or spoilt hay. Abortions occur in late gestation. Diagnosis is based on the identification of the causal organism and the placental lesions which are similar to those associated with fungal agents (see below).
- *Actinomyces pyogenes* is a common cause of sporadic abortion at any time but usually in late gestation. Although a common secondary invader to other primary pathogens, it is likely that when identified its presence is significant. Diagnosis is based on the isolation of the organism from the fetus or fetal membranes.
- *Listeria monocytogenes* causes sporadic, late abortion and may follow a bout of pyrexia. Diagnosis is based upon identifying the organism in direct smears or using immunofluorescence and the presence of yellow/grey necrotic foci on the fetal liver and cotyledons. It is often associated with the feeding of silage.

- There are two subspecies of *Campylobacter fetus*, namely *venerealis* and *fetus*. The former subspecies is venereally transmitted and usually exerts its effect upon reproduction by preventing fertilisation or causing embryonic death (see section 8.2); however, abortions at 6–8 months can occur. Subspecies *fetus* is not transmitted venereally and can cause sporadic abortion from 4 months of gestation. Diagnosis can be made by identification of the organism by direct smear or culture, use of fluorescent antibodies, vaginal mucus agglutination tests, or serology. Infection associated with *C. fetus venerealis* is self-limiting because most infected cows become immune in 3–6 months; since it is transmitted venereally, AI using antibiotic-treated semen from a bull known to be free from infection should be used.
- *Brucella abortus* is a major cause of abortion worldwide as well as being an important zoonosis. Abortion occurs usually at 6–9 months of gestation, but earlier abortions can occur as well as stillborn and live weakly calves. Infection usually occurs following the ingestion of food contaminated with fetal membranes or genital discharges from infected cows that have aborted, or calved. Diagnosis is made following the identification of the organism in stained smears from contaminated material, culture, fluorescent antibody tests, colony blot ELISA and a variety of serological tests on milk, serum, vaginal mucus and semen. The disease can be controlled by vaccination using S19 live antigen and killed cultures of S45/20 or in the long term by identification of affected animals and slaughter.
- *Escherichia coli*.
- Fungi are a common cause of abortion at 4–9 months of gestation. Usually sporadic in nature and due mainly to *Aspergillus* sp. and *Mucor* sp. Diagnosis can frequently be made on the typical ringworm-like lesions on the integument of the fetus, the necrotic placentitis and leathery intercotyledonary allantochorion, and the presence of fungal hyphae. Mouldy forage and bedding should not be used.
- *Tritrichomonas fetus* infection mainly results in infertility (see section 8.2); however, the flagellated protozoan can result in early abortion at <4 months of gestation. The disease is venereal. Diagnosis is based on the identification of the organism in the fetus or discharges from the genital tract; it can also be identified in preputial washings of infected bulls. Vaginal and uterine mucus can be collected to identify agglutinating antibodies. Control is based upon the fact that most cows become immune after several months and that bulls, although they can be cured, are likely to be permanent carriers of the infection. Thus AI using semen from clean bulls is preferable to prevent spread to non-immune animals.
- *Neosporum caninum* is a protozoan which in recent years has been shown to cause abortion from about 6 months of gestation; it can reach epizootic proportions. The organism, which causes nervous disease in dogs, can be diagnosed by the identification of specific lesions in the brain of aborted fetuses and by an immunofluorescent antibody test in

blood from cows that have aborted. Prevention of dogs contaminating cattle food must assist in the control of the disease. It is likely to be identified as a major cause of abortion in cattle in the future.

- The togavirus that causes *bovine viral diarrhoea (BVD)* can cause abortion as well as embryonic death (see section 8.2) and can also result in stillbirths and weakly live calves, sometimes with congenital defects. Abortion is preceded by a mild, transient disease which goes undetected or an obvious febrile disease. Diagnosis is based upon the identification of gross and microscopic lesions in the fetus, virus isolation, a fluorescent antibody test, or serological tests. Control involves culling of persistently infected animals, introduction of only immune or disease-free animals into the herd, and vaccination.
- *Bovine herpes virus (BHV-1)* infection can cause sporadic abortions or abortion storms with up to 60% of cows affected. It also causes embryonic death (see section 8.2). Abortions, which occur at 4–9 months of gestation, may or may not be preceded by other clinical signs of the disease, such as respiratory disease. Diagnosis is based upon fetal lesions, virus isolation, fluorescent antibody test on fetal tissue, or serological tests. Control involves isolation and vaccination.
- Catarrhal vaginocervicitis due to an enterovirus.
- Parainfluenza 3 virus.
- *Chlamydia psittaci* causes abortion at 7–9 months of gestation.
- *Mycoplasma bovis, Acholeplasma laidlawii* and other mycoplasma species cause infertility, vulvovaginal lesions and abortion.
- *Haemophilus somnus* causes abortion but also lesions of the tubular genital tract which result in infertility.
- *Coxiella burnetii* – a zoonosis.

Non-infectious causes of abortion

These are essentially the same as those listed in sections 7.7 and 8.2.

- Congenital abnormalities due to genetic factors or teratogens.
- Endocrine deficiencies and excesses.
- Poisonous plants.
- Toxic substances, such as nitrates, mycotoxins, warfarin, goitrogens.
- Nutritional deficiencies, e.g. vitamin A, iodine.
- Nutritional excesses, e.g. high protein diets.
- Heat stress.
- Therapeutic substances, e.g. prostaglandin $F_2\alpha$ or analogues, oestrogens, corticosteroids.

8.8   DIAGNOSIS OF CAUSES OF ABORTION

Identification of a specific cause of abortion is frequently difficult and, as a consequence, the diagnostic success rate is low (< 7–8%). This is due to:

- A delay between the causal agent exerting its effect and expulsion of the fetus.
- Autolysis of the fetus and fetal membranes.
- Absence of pathognomonic lesions.
- Unavailability of a diagnostic test.
- Inadequate or incorrect material submitted to the laboratory.

To assist in the detailed investigation of abortions (other than that required under the Brucellosis Orders, see section 8.6), the following procedure should be followed:

- Obtain an accurate date of natural service or AI, when evidence of growth retardation can be determined by comparing fetal weight and dimensions with calculated gestation length.
- Obtain details of husbandry changes, milk yield and health status during previous weeks, including other abortions, stillbirths or weak live calves.
- Examine fetus and fetal membranes for evidence of specific lesions.
- Submit the whole fetus (where possible) and fetal membranes to the laboratory as soon as possible. Refrigerate if there is a possible delay.
- If not the whole fetus, then the following should be collected and submitted: 2ml of abomasal contents and thoracic or abdominal fluid (if present) collected with a sterile needle with syringe or vacutainer; large portion of fresh lung, liver, kidney, spleen and salivary gland; fresh cotyledon; formalin-fixed lung, liver, heart and cotyledon; 7 ml of clotted dam's blood repeated 2–3 weeks later.

8.9 STILLBIRTH

Stillbirth is defined as the birth of a dead calf after 272 days of gestation. Most stillbirths occur during the act of parturition.

8.10 FETAL MACERATION

This occurs as a consequence of fetal death, usually in mid-to-late gestation. There is regression of the CL, and dilation of the cervix, but the fetus is not aborted and remains in the genital tract. Bacteria enter through the dilated cervix causing putrefaction which together with autolytic change, results in digestion of the fetal tissues, ultimately leaving only the fetal skeleton. Since treatment with hormones, such as prostaglandin $F_2\alpha$ or oestrogens, is not effective, the only method of removing the macerated tissue is by hysterotomy. Access to the uterus through a laparotomy incision is difficult and subsequent fertility will be poor.

8.11 CONGENITAL ABNORMALITIES

These are abnormalities of structure or function that are present before birth or at the time of birth. In some cases they may not be apparent until some time after birth. The consequences are:

- They may cause prenatal death (see sections 7.3, 8.1, 8.3 and 8.4).
- They may cause dystocia (see section 9.8).
- They may adversely affect the ability of the calf to survive after birth.
- It may be uneconomic to retain the calf because it may not be normally productive, or it may transmit the defect to its progeny.
- They may develop a disease such as BSE, which may have been transmitted *in utero*.

About 1% of calves have congenital defects.

Causes

- Environmental factors such as heat stress causing hyperthermia or teratogenic agents.
- Genetic defects due to gene mutations or chromosome abnormalities.
- Infectious agents such as BVD, bluetongue virus or Akabane virus.

In many cases a precise cause is not known. Therefore any congenital defect should be treated as possibly genetic in origin; the calf should not be retained for breeding purposes.

Some common congenital abnormalities and their causes

- Major abnormalities
  Schistosoma reflexus: cause unknown (see Fig. 8.2).
  Conjoined twins: cause unknown (see Fig. 8.3).
  Achondroplasia: genetic (see Fig. 8.4).
- Skeletal and muscular abnormalities
  Hydrocephalus: genetic.
  Torticollis and scoliosis (deviation and twisting of vertebral column): possibly genetic.
  Cleft palate: genetic and teratogenic.
  Arthrogryposis (joint flexion and fusion): genetic and teratogenic.
  Agenesis of the tail: unknown.
  Shortening of lower jaw: unknown.
  Polydactyly (additional digits or limbs): unknown.
  Syndactyly (fusion of functional digits): genetic.
  Double muscling: genetic.
  Contracted flexor tendons: genetic (see Fig. 8.5).
- Abnormalities of the eye
  Microphthalmia: cause unknown.
  Dermoid: genetic.
  Cataract: genetic.

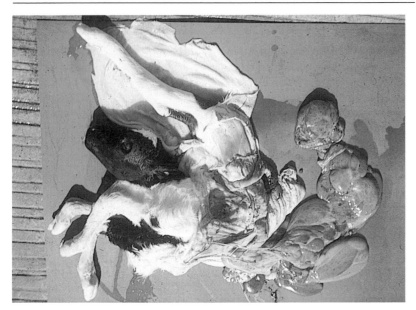

Fig. 8.2. Schistosoma reflexus calf.

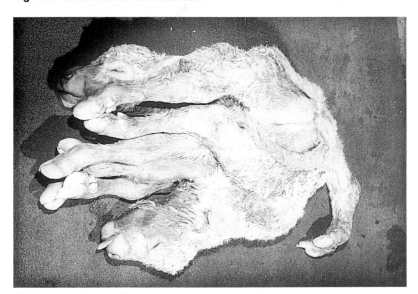

Fig. 8.3. Conjoined Charolais twins at term.

- Cardiovascular defects
  Ectopic heart: possibly genetic.
  Patent ductus arteriosus and foramen ovale: cause unknown.
- Cutaneous system
  Epitheliogenesis imperfecta: genetic.
  Umbilical hernia: genetic.

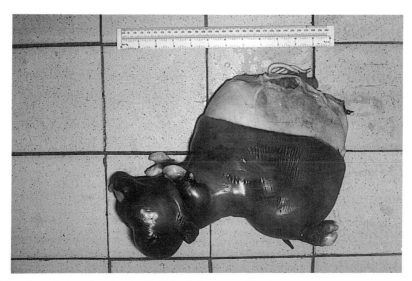

Fig. 8.4. Achondroplastic (bulldog) Dexter calf.

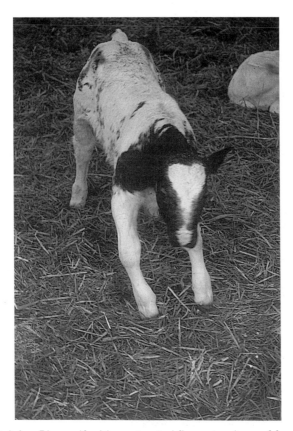

Fig. 8.5. Belgian Blue calf with contracted flexor tendons of forelimbs.

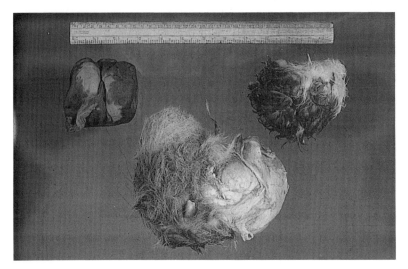

Fig. 8.6. Examples of three fetal moles (amorphous globosus).

- Defects of the genital system (see sections 3.5 and 7.6).
- Fetal moles/amorphous globosus (see Fig. 8.6).

8.12 CERVICO-VAGINAL PROLAPSE

This implies the protrusion of the vagina and cervix through the vulva. The severity varies from slight and intermittent protrusion of the floor of the vagina, to the severe with permanent protrusion of the vagina and cervix.

Causes

Prolapse is essential due to weakness of the constrictor muscles of the vestibule and vulva and perhaps the stretching of the suspensory ligaments of the genital tract. Several factors predispose to the condition:

- Genetic: most frequently seen in beef breeds such as the Hereford and Charolais.
- Obesity: especially due to extensive deposition of retroperitoneal fat.
- Pregnancy: most frequently seen in late pregnancy, therefore it might be associated with relaxation of the vagina and perineum due to the endocrine status of the cow.
- High roughage feeding: increased rumen size so that there is increased intra-abdominal pressure.
- Self-perpetuation: as the prolapse develops the mucosa becomes progressively more dehydrated, devitalised, traumatised and infected, thus stimulating the cow to strain.

Diagnosis and prognosis

The condition is usually obvious on visual inspection. Vaginal polyps and protruding fetal membranes could cause a misdiagnosis initially.

A mild degree of prolapse a few weeks before calving is of little consequence; more severe prolapse, especially if it occurs 6 or more weeks before term, must be treated. Failure to do so will result in breakdown of the cervical mucus seal, bacterial invasion of the uterus, fetal death and abortion.

Treatment

The main aim should be the retention of the prolapsed tissues until the cow calves, when the problem will usually be resolved. As there is a strong possibility that prolapse will recur in the next and succeeding pregnancies it is doubtful if the cow should be bred from again. There is also a chance that the tendency may be inherited.

Caudal epidural anaesthesia is induced to abolish straining, the mucosa is cleansed with non-irritant fluid (preferably physiological saline or water), dried, anointed with petroleum jelly or other emollient agent, gently replaced and retained in place by one of the following methods:

- Rope truss.
- Vulval sutures such as simple mattress or quill sutures.
- Perivulval, subcutaneous suture using nylon tape – Bühner method, which is the method of choice (see Fig. 8.7).
- Caslick operation.

The temporary sutures must be removed at calving and in many cases parturition should be induced (see section 3.12). Permanent methods such as sub-mucous resection or cervico-vaginal fixation can be used, but these latter methods are difficult.

8.13 UTERINE TORSION

Most cases of uterine torsion occur at the time of calving (see section 9.9); a small number of cows develop uterine torsion during late pregnancy. It is likely that that there will be clinical signs only when it exceeds 180° about the longitudinal axis.

When there is abdominal pain or discomfort in late pregnancy with elevated pulse rate, uterine torsion should be considered as a possible cause. Diagnosis can be made by vaginal palpation (unless it is a heifer) or rectal palpation. Correction is by rolling the cow, or via a laparotomy and perhaps hysterotomy (see section 9.8). In some cases fetal death with mummification or uterine rupture with a pseudo-ectopic pregnancy can occur.

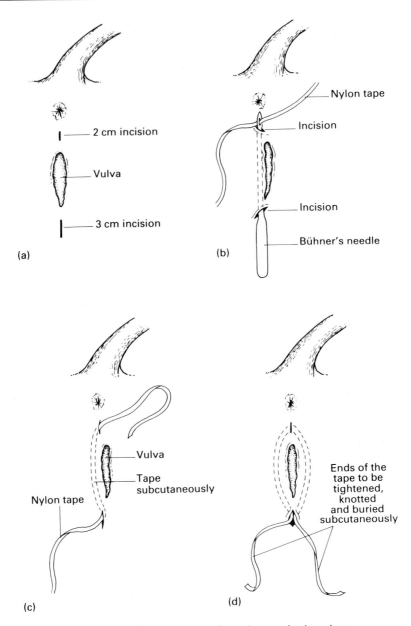

Fig. 8.7. Bühner method for retention of cervico-vaginal prolapse.

8.14 UTERINE RUPTURE

This can occur spontaneously during pregnancy for no apparent reason or as a consequence of uterine torsion (see section 8.13). The fetus can die or in some cases, provided that the umbilicus and placenta are intact, it will develop as a pseudo-ectopic pregnancy.

8.15 HYDROPS AMNII AND HYDROPS ALLANTOIS

The normal volumes of amniotic and allantoic fluid during pregnancy are given in section 2.5. Hydrops implies excess production of the fetal fluids – hydrops allantois is by far the most common of the two. Slight to moderate excess fetal fluids can pass unnoticed; however, in severe cases the volume of amniotic fluid can reach 100 l and allantoic fluid 250 l.

- *Clinical signs.* In the last third of gestation there will be evidence of excess abdominal distension. There will be reduced appetite because the rumen is compressed and becomes small. The cow will have difficulty walking and, if symptoms are severe, will remain recumbent.
- *Diagnosis* is made on history and clinical signs. Abdominal percussion will reveal a large fluid-filled mass and rectal examination will reveal a grossly enlarged uterus where few caruncles can be palpated.
- *Prognosis* is grave unless the cow is close to term when it will calve spontaneously, or is treated. Dystocia due to uterine inertia (see section 9.9) or retained placenta followed by metritis are highly likely (see section 11.8).
- *Treatment.* Unless the cow is valuable, treatment is rarely economic and thus slaughter is in most cases preferable. Parturition can be induced with corticosteroids (see section 3.12) or alternatively a hysterotomy can be performed to remove the calf; however, the fetal fluids must be allowed to escape slowly over a period of about 30 min. This ensures that circulatory shock does not occur due to splanchnic pooling, if the fluid is allowed to escape suddenly with a sudden reduction in intra-abdominal pressure.

9 Dystocia

9.1 DEFINITION

Dystocia is defined as difficult birth. It may range from a slight delay in the process to the complete inability of the cow to give birth. Consequences of dystocia are important and may be:

- a dead or weakly live calf;
- reduced appetite, milk yield and hence overall production;
- reduced fertility;
- sterility;
- a dead cow.

9.2 INCIDENCE

It is difficult to give a meaningful overall figure because it is influenced by such factors as the age and parity of the dam, the breed of the sire and the breed of dam. Figures of between 3% and 8% are frequently quoted, whilst in breeds where muscular hypertrophy occurs, such as the Belgian Blue, up to 80% has been reported.

9.3 CAUSES

Traditionally these are divided into those that are primarily of maternal origin and those that are primarily of fetal origin. Frequently the distinction is not clear and one problem may give rise to another.

9.4 DEALING WITH A CASE OF DYSTOCIA

A suspected dystocia case should always be treated as an emergency, requiring a visit and examination as soon as possible. The ultimate aim should be a live cow and calf.

A detailed history should be obtained:

- Age and parity of the cow.
- Previous calving history.
- Health during pregnancy, especially in immediate period.
- Present appetite and activity.
- Date of service or expected calving date.
- Sire of calf and details of other calvings where he was the sire.
- First signs of impending calving (onset of first stage) (see section 3.8).
- Evidence of straining, when it was first seen and its nature.
- Evidence of fetus and/or fetal membrane at the vulva.
- Evidence of rupture of allantochorion or amnion with escape of fluids.
- The nature of any examination or attempted delivery by farm personnel.

9.5 CLINICAL EXAMINATION

The cow should be adequately restrained in a suitable calving box (see section 3.11). The following procedure should be followed:

- Assess generally the cow's bodily condition and health, with particular emphasis on the presence of hypocalcaemia or mastitis.
- Assess the vulva and pelvic ligaments for degree of relaxation.
- Note the nature of any vulval discharges, particularly their smell.
- Examine the vulva for evidence of trauma from previous interferences.
- Thoroughly wash the peritoneum and vulva with warm water, soap or surgical scrub.
- Insert a clean (preferably sleeved) adequately lubricated arm gently into the vagina. The presence of a calf (or calves) should be determined together with its disposition.
- Assess the presence of a live calf by eliciting flexor, eye or suck reflexes and note a heart beat or carotid pulse. In posterior presentation the anal reflex can be assessed.
- Assess the integrity of the amnion and allantochorion.
- Note the degree of dilatation of the cervix. When it is fully dilated only a small frill of tissue separating the vagina from the uterus can be palpated.
- Note whether the calf is in the abdomen or the pelvic canal.
- Determine and report the presence of any lacerations, haematomas or other injuries. *
- After vaginal delivery of a calf *always* check whether there is another one.

9.6 DIAGNOSIS

The history followed by clinical examination should enable a diagnosis of dystocia to be made. The following is a reminder of the durations of the stages:

- First stage should be completed by 6 h; heifers frequently require longer.
- Second stage usually takes about 70 min; it should certainly be completed by 4 h except in heifers where up to 6 h should be given to enable adequate dilation of the birth canal.

9.7 TREATMENT

Treatment will depend upon the precise cause of the dystocia; however, the following general techniques are frequently used.

Correction of faulty disposition

During the first stage of parturition (see section 3.8) the calf undergoes changes in its disposition within the uterus so that it can readily pass through the birth canal. These changes involve extension of the extremities and rotation of the calf about its longitudinal axis so that its dorsal surface is adjacent to the sacrum and vertebrae of the cow. Whether the calf enters the birth canal anterioraly or posteriorly is determined early in gestation.

The normal disposition of the calf can be described as follows: *anterior longitudinal presentation* (the relationship of the longitudinal axis of the calf to the birth canal), *dorsal position* (the relationship of the dorsal surface of the calf to the sacrum and vertebrae of the dam) and *extended posture* (the head and limbs are extended) (See Fig. 9.1).

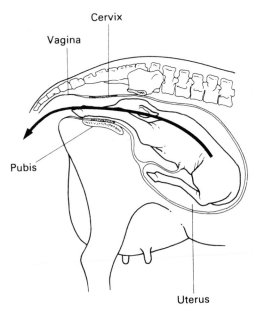

Fig. 9.1. Calf in normal disposition for birth – anterior longitudinal presentation, dorsal position, extended posture. (Arrow indicates arc-like passage of calf from uterus to exterior.)

The calf must be in normal disposition before it can be expelled. This is achieved by applying corrective forces *per vaginum* and is largely dependent upon simple mechanical procedures. Correction is facilitated by repelling the calf back into the uterus to provide sufficient space to perform the necessary manipulation. B_2 mimetic agents, such as clenbuterol hydrochloride, relax the uterus, and caudal epidural anaesthesia prevents straining and facilitates repulsion. Correction of faulty disposition is easier if the calf is alive (because spontaneous movements occur) and if there is adequate natural or supplementary lubrication.

Traction

This is required to supplement the normal expulsive forces which are a combination of myometrial contractions and abdominal straining. It is required when the expulsive force is insufficient to expel the calf and preferably should be coordinated with the straining. Traction is applied through rope snares or obstetrical chains which are placed behind the ears and occiput in the case of head snares (see Fig. 9.2a) or above the fetlock joint in the case of the limbs (see Fig. 9.2b). There must be adequate lubrication, either natural from fetal fluids or artificial in the form of cellulose obstetrical lubricants or soap.

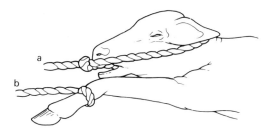

Fig. 9.2. Sites of attachment of rope snares for traction. (a) Benesch snare for traction to head. (b) Limb snare for traction to limbs.

Traction must be applied in such a direction as to simulate the normal progression of the calf through the birth canal (see Fig. 9.1) with one foot slightly in advance of the other. Excessive traction should not be applied to the head. The direction of the force follows an arc and is dependent upon the situation of the calf relative to the birth canal.

Instruments used in traction, such as 'calf-pullers', 'calving jacks' or pulley blocks, must be used with great care because of the mechanical advantage generated and should only be used by experienced and responsible persons. Inappropriate use can cause damage to the cow and calf.

Fetotomy (embryotomy)

This technique involves the amputation of a part of the calf, or its division into portions so that they can be extracted *per vaginum*. The following basic principles must be followed:

- The calf must be dead or worthless, i.e. fetal monster, in which case it must be killed before the procedure commences.
- Caudal epidural anaesthesia should be used.
- Fetotomy should rarely involve more than one cut.
- A proper instrument should be used.
- The technique must be performed as aseptically as possible.

Most fetotomes are of the tubular type (see Fig. 9.3) which protect the cow's genital tract from trauma. Cutting is done with a braided steel wire which is passed around the part of the calf to be cut.

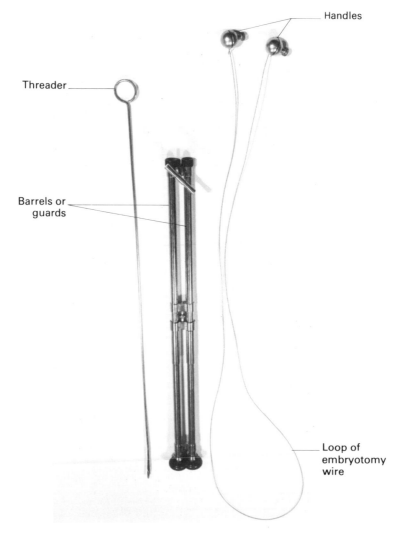

Handles

Threader

Barrels or guards

Loop of embryotomy wire

Fig. 9.3. Thygesen's tubular fetotome.

Fetotomy must be performed with care since trauma, particularly if the procedure is extensive and prolonged, can affect the fertility of the cow.

Caesarean operation

This is the method of choice when a normal, live calf is present and dystocia cannot be corrected by any other means. Provided that it is performed properly there should be a high calf survival rate and low cow mortality rate, with a minimal reduction in fertility.

Details of the technique may be found in standard textbooks on bovine surgery.

9.8 SPECIFIC CAUSES OF DYSTOCIA – GROUP 1

The first group of specific causes of dystocia are those where the cow is observed to have had forceful, but unproductive, straining for several hours.

Feto-maternal disproportion

This implies that the fetus is larger than normal or that the birth canal, particularly the bony pelvis, is too small or of bad conformation. In both cases the calf is incapable of passing through the birth canal without assistance.

This is the commonest cause of dystocia attended by veterinarians; it is especially common in heifers and beef breeds with muscular hypertrophy (see section 8.11).

There is a *history* of unproductive straining, perhaps with the extremity of one or two limbs protruding from the vulva.

Clinical examination per vaginum will show that the calf is in normal presentation, position and posture (see section 9.7) with the cervix fully dilated and the vagina, vulva and perineum normally relaxed.

Treatment in the first instance will be by attempted traction, provided that there is adequate lubrication. Treatment can frequently be assessed subjectively by determining progress after a trial period of 10 min of coordinated effort by three persons. Traction is likely to be successful if the calf is in anterior presentation so that traction allows both elbows to pass over the brim of the pelvis together. Alternatively, attempts can be made to predict the success of traction by using Hindson's formula to calculate the traction ratio (TR):

$$TR = \frac{\text{Interischial distance}}{\text{Calf digital diameter}} \times \frac{P_1}{P_2} \times \frac{1}{E}$$

P_1 = Parity factor of 0.95 for heifers
P_2 = Correction factor for posterior presentation of 1.05
E = Factor of 1.05 for breeds with muscular hypertrophy

TRs of 2.5 or more are likely to be successfully resolved by traction; TRs of 2.5 or less require a caesarean.

In some cases, traction successfully delivers the calf to the level of the chest but the caudal part of the calf will not traverse the birth canal. This is referred to as 'hip lock', where the greater trochanters of the calf's femur impinge upon the shafts of the ileum and the stifles impinge upon the pelvic brim. The calf should be repelled and rotated through 45° to 90° about its longitudinal axis and traction repeated. Failure will require fetotomy (see section 9.7).

A caesarean operation is the method of choice if traction is unsuccessful. It is preferable to choose this method if the calf is alive, rather than to fail with excessive traction and produce a dead calf.

Fetotomy is the only feasible method of treatment following 'hip lock' when the calf is dead. The cranial portion of the calf is amputated; it is eviscerated and the pelvis bisected using the fetotome. Each portion is removed separately.

Prevention of feto-maternal disproportion is the aim and this can be achieved as follows:

- Dam selection – ensure that she is of adequate size.
- Sire selection – do not use breeds of bulls with a high predisposition to causing dystocia. Select sires with a low dystocia rate for heifers.
- Ensure that cows are not overfed and hence become over-fat. Reduced food intake has little or no effect upon fetal growth rate and size.
- Induce calving before term (see section 3.12).
- Select cows with good pelvic conformation. The pelvis should slope cranio-caudally with wide hook and pin bones.

Partial (or incomplete) cervical dilatation

There is a *history* of unproductive straining (for exceptions see section 9.9).

Clinical examination per vaginum will identify a partially dilated cervix with part of the calf (usually one or both limbs and perhaps part of the head) protruding through it; in some cases the cervix feels like a tight band of tissue.

It is *caused by* hypocalcaemia, fibrosis of the cervix, endocrine deficiencies, or failure of the cervical tissue to respond to the endocrine changes that occur at the time of parturition.

Treatment. If the calf is alive give calcium borogluconate intravenously and wait for 1 h in case the first stage has not been completed. If there is no response after this time, gentle traction might complete dilatation if it is nearly complete; alternatively a caesarean operation is indicated. A dead and putrefying calf is frequently associated with a long-standing dystocia due to some other reason, so that the cervix, having dilated normally, has started to close.

Vulval or vaginal stricture

There is a *history* of unproductive straining, usually in a heifer.

Clinical examination in the case of vulval stricture will show a small, poorly relaxed vulva into which it is difficult to insert a hand and arm. One or both feet may protrude from the vulva and the calf is in normal presentation, position and posture. The cervix is fully dilated. Where there is a vaginal stricture this will be identified as a stenosis on vaginal exploration.

It is *caused by* an endocrine abnormality, failure of the tissues to respond to the endocrine changes associated with parturition, or a congenital defect; it may be indicative of a premature calving or late term abortion (see sections 8.5–8.7).

Treatment of vulval stricture is by gentle traction with adequate lubrication to stretch the vulva, or an episiotomy (see Fig. 11.2) or a β_2 mimetic drug such as clenbuterol to postpone calving and thus allow time for softening of the vulva (see section 3.13). Traction can lead to 1°, 2° or 3° perineal lacerations (see section 11.2). Vaginal strictures if slight can be dealt with by careful traction or an episiotomy at 10 and 2 o'clock to prevent a third degree perineal laceration occurring (see section 11.2); a severe stricture requires a caesarean operation.

Soft tissue obstructions

There is a *history* of unproductive straining.

Clinical examination per vaginum will show the calf in normal presentation, position and posture; the cervix will be fully dilated, but there will be a soft tissue obstruction which might be confused with vaginal stricture (above). There may be a vaginal tumour, remnants of Müllerian ducts present as fibrous tissue bands or a double cervix with the calf's extremities entering both cervical canals.

Treatment. Müllerian duct remnants can be cut with scissors. Tumours and double cervix require a caesarean operation.

Bony defects of the pelvis

There is a *history* of unproductive straining and possibly previous injury to the pelvis.

Clinical examination may show external signs of a pelvic defect such as sacro-iliac dislocation. Vaginal examination will show the calf in normal presentation, position and posture, with a fully dilated cervix and a deformed and abnormal bony birth canal.

Treatment. If it is a slight defect careful traction can be tried; otherwise, perform a caesarean operation and do not breed from the cow again.

Uterine torsion (see also section 9.9)

There is a *history* of some evidence of mild unproductive straining, although in many cases there will be no such evidence. The cow will often stand with her tail elevated and showing signs of discomfort.

Clinical examination of the vulva and perineum may show slight distortion, loss of symmetry and pulling into the pelvis. It will be difficult to explore the vagina manually if the torsion is 360° because the lumen will be almost occluded. If torsion is 180° or less, it is generally possible to insert the arm into the vagina and through the cervix by following the direction of the twist. Torsions can be to the right or left; the latter are more common. The calf's limbs may be involved in the torsion.

The *cause* of the condition is not known for certain; it is probably associated with vigorous fetal movements, perhaps stimulated by the onset of uterine contraction of the first stage of parturition (see section 3.8), and the unstable suspension of the gravid uterus, especially in pluriparous animals.

Treatment. The simplest, most successful method is to roll the cow. She is cast, her fore limbs and hind limbs are hobbled and she is placed in lateral recumbency on the side to which the uterus is twisted (i.e. on her left side if left-sided torsion). An arm is inserted into the vagina to grasp the fetus if possible or at least to try to stop the uterus moving; the cow is then suddenly and rapidly turned through 180°. If it is successful the torsion will be felt to unwind; if it is not, or if it is only partially corrected, rolling should be repeated.

In most cases once the torsion has been corrected the cervix will be found to be dilated and the calf can be delivered by traction. If the cervix is not fully dilated the cow should be left for 1 h to allow dilatation to occur. If it fails to occur, a caesarean operation will be necessary.

If rolling fails to correct the torsion it can be treated via a left flank laparotomy and if this is unsuccessful by a caesarean operation.

Simultaneous presentation of twins

There is a *history* of unproductive straining, perhaps with one or more limb extremities appearing at the vulva.

Clinical examination shows a normal, relaxed vulva and perineum, a fully dilated cervix and two calves entering the birth canal simultaneously. Careful palpation must be used to determine the relationships of the various extremities and the disposition of the calves. For the possibility of conjoined twins see 'Monsters' below.

Treatment. One calf should be repelled to provide space for the other to be drawn into the birth canal. It is often difficult to match pairs of limbs with the appropriate torso. If both calves are equally placed in the birth canal and one is in posterior longitudinal presentation, it should be delivered first. If one is in advance of the other then this one should be delivered first.

Twin calves are usually smaller than singletons and hence manipulation is easier.

Monsters (congenitally deformed calves)

There is a *history* of unproductive straining, perhaps with extremities protruding from the vulva; in the case of schistosoma reflexus (see below), intestines and other viscera may be at the vulva.

Clinical examination per vaginum will reveal a normal relaxed vulva, fully dilated cervix and parts of the calf in the birth canal. It is frequently difficult to ascertain the type of monster.

Causes of congenital abnormalities giving rise to monsters are described in section 8.11, together with illustrations of examples.

The following are some of the more common types of abnormalities:

- *Schistosoma reflexus* (see section 8.11 and Fig. 8.2). It will either be in visceral presentation, when the intestines protrude into the vagina and even through the vulva, or the limbs are presented. When they are small, delivery via the vagina is possible; otherwise caesarean operation or fetotomy is necessary.
- *Conjoined twins* (see Fig. 8.3). Fusion of the two calves can be at virtually any point of the body. Differentiation from normal twins can sometimes be difficult (see above). They must be delivered by caesarean operation.
- *Perosomus elumbis.* This is where the cranial part of the body is normal but the caudal part has ankylosis of the vertebrae and hind limbs. It is sometimes difficult to identify on vaginal examination, and should be delivered by caesarean operation.
- Arthrogryposis, torticollis and scoliosis describe conditions where the extremities are flexed and rigid. They can be difficult to determine until it is found impossible to extend the extremities by manipulation *per vaginum*. Delivery is following fetotomy or caesarean operation; in the case of the latter, partial fetotomy may be required through the hysterotomy incision.
- *Ascites.* This is sometimes seen in association with achondroplasia or dwarfism. Treat by draining the abdomen and traction, or by caesarean operation (see Fig. 8.4).
- *Anasarca.* This is generalised subcutaneous oedema, and is treated by caesarean operation.

Abnormal disposition

This is the commonest cause of dystocia in all types and breeds of cattle.

Clinical signs. There is unproductive straining, perhaps with some evidence of fetal extremities at the vulva. Vaginal examination will show a fully dilated cervix with the calf in abnormal presentation, position or posture. Careful palpation will enable the precise abnormality to be determined.

The *cause* of abnormal disposition is not fully understood. Some of the following may be involved: failure of development of reflexes in the calf, inadequate stimulation of fetal movement, fetal anoxia.

Treatment. General principles are covered in section 9.7.

Abnormal disposition due to postural abnormalities

These abnormalities can be unilateral or bilateral, involving the head and neck or limbs alone, or in combination.

Postural abnormalities occurring with the calf in *anterior presentation* are:

- Unilateral or bilateral carpal flexion; treated by repulsion and extension.
- Unilateral or bilateral elbow flexion; treated by repulsion and extension.
- Unilateral or bilateral shoulder flexion; treated by repulsion and extension. The head can protrude from the vulva and become oedematous, congested and enlarged ('hung calf'). If it is dead, simple fetotomy involving amputation of the head by disarticulation of the atlanto-occipital joint allows repulsion and extension of the fore limbs.
- Lateral flexion of the head and neck; this can also occur with other postural abnormalities. Treatment is by repulsion and extension unless there is ankylosis of the vertebrae. Fetotomy or caesarean operation should be performed if this is unsuccessful.
- Ventral flexion of the head and neck, treated by repulsion and extension.
- Hip flexion ('dog-sitting' posture) where the hind limbs are extended towards the calf's head and are placed over the pelvic brim of the cow into the birth canal; it can be confused with simultaneous presentation of twins (see above). Treatment is by repulsion and traction.

Postural abnormalities occurring with the calf in *posterior presentation* are:

- Unilateral or bilateral hock flexion; treated by repulsion and extension.
- Unilateral or bilateral hip flexion ('breech posture'); treated by repulsion and extension.

Abnormal disposition due to positional abnormalities

These abnormalities can occur with the calf in anterior or posterior longitudinal presentation in combination with abnormalities of posture. These include:

- Ventral position.
- Left lateral position.
- Right lateral position.
- Variations between, e.g. ventro-lateral position.

Treatment involves repulsion and rotation about the longitudinal axis, which may need to be repeated several times until correction is complete. Adequate lubrication is important.

Abnormal disposition due to presentational abnormalities

These abnormalities are not common in the cow unless posterior longitudinal presentation is considered abnormal (about 5% of calves are born thus, frequently without dystocia). Feto-maternal disproportion is accentuated in this presentation and the incidence of stillbirth is higher than following anterior presentation.

Transverse presentations are rare because of the shape of the gravid uterus and restricted space.

9.9 SPECIFIC CAUSES OF DYSTOCIA – GROUP 2

These are where there is no – or limited – evidence of straining, and the first stage of parturition (see section 3.8) is apparently prolonged.

Uterine rupture (see section 11.6)
There is a *history* of some unproductive straining which has now ceased, or there has been some evidence of the onset of the first stage of parturition without progression to the second stage. The clinical signs will depend upon when the rupture occurred.

Clinical examination per vaginum will show a dilated or partially dilated cervix with no calf palpable and evidence of a uterine tear through which the umbilicus passes.

Treatment is by laparotomy.

Uterine torsion
See section 9.8. This can occur without any evidence of straining but with a history of the cow being in the first stage of parturition without progression to the second stage.

Incomplete cervical dilatation
See section 9.8.

There is a *history* of a prolonged first stage with no progression to the second stage; there is no evidence of straining.

Clinical examination per vaginum will identify that the cervix is only partially dilated and is insufficient to allow the passage of the calf's extremities; fetal membranes may be protruding. Assess the viability of the calf and look for signs of putrefactive changes.

Treatment. It is possible that the cow has not completed first stage; therefore leave her for at least 1 h and re-examine for evidence of further dilatation. Calcium borogluconate should be given intravenously even if there are no clinical signs of milk fever. If dilatation fails to occur the calf must be delivered by a caesarean operation (see section 9.7).

If the calf is dead and there are signs of putrefaction it is probably due to failure of expulsion of the calf, so that the cervix has now closed. It occurs following late abortions (see sections 8.7 and 8.8).

Uterine inertia
Primary uterine inertia is quite common especially in old, pluriparous cows; it is also associated with late abortions (see sections 8.7 and 8.8) and hypocalcaemia.

There is a *history* of a prolonged first stage, with no signs of straining. There may be some evidence of hypocalcaemia.

Clinical examination per vaginum shows a fully dilated cervix with fetal membranes entering the birth canal but with the calf in normal disposition still within the uterus.

Treatment. Calcium borogluconate should be given and, provided the vulva and vagina are relaxed, the calf delivered by traction.

Ventral deviation or displacement of the uterus

This is not a common condition.

The *history* is of an old pluriparous cow with pendulous abdomen, perhaps with rupture of the rectus muscles or a prepubic tendon, in prolonged first stage with no signs of straining.

Clinical examination per vaginum will show a fully dilated cervix with the calf present in the uterus and situated deep in the abdomen. There may be some evidence of uterine inertia.

Treatment. Give calcium borogluconate and use traction.

10   Placental Retention

10.1   INTRODUCTION

The placenta is normally shed about 6 h, on average, after the expulsion of the calf. The method of normal separation and expulsion has been described in section 3.10.

10.2   INCIDENCE

It is difficult to obtain accurate figures for this because of varying opinion on the normal time for separation and expulsion. However, it is more prevalent in dairy cows than in beef cows – an average figure would be about 8%. It is more prevalent following certain abnormalities (see below), and on certain farms in certain years there is a dramatic increase. Very often the cause is unknown.

10.3   CAUSES

These are not fully understood and frequently no precise explanation can be found.

- *Failure of placental maturation.* This is the most important cause of placental retention. The endocrine changes responsible for the initiation of parturition (see section 3.6) are also involved in the maturational changes in the placenta.
- *Premature birth* – either abortion (see sections 8.7 and 8.8) or following induction of parturition (see section 3.12). This may result from incomplete placental maturation.
- *Uterine inertia.* Physical detachment of the placenta is dependent upon the persistence of uterine contractions after the expulsion of the calf (see section 5.4). Factors such as hypocalcaemia, which depresses myometrial activity, dystocia, which may result in secondary uterine inertia (see section 9.9), and endocrine deficiencies or imbalances, can all

influence the strength and duration of uterine contractions. However, whilst this may result in a delay of the final expulsion of the placenta, it is unlikely to cause true long lasting retention.

- *Twins and multiple births.* Retention might be due to a slight premature birth since gestation length for twins is shorter, or to uterine inertia due to over-stretching of the myometrium.
- *Pathological placental lesions*, such as placentitis, oedema of villi and crypts, or necrosis of villi, may increase the degree of physical attachment or prevent separation.

10.4   CONSEQUENCES

It is difficult to quantify these accurately because placental retention may be a manifestation of some other reproductive abnormality. However, they can be listed as:

- Tainted milk flavour (it should be discarded).
- Possibly reduced appetite and milk yield.
- Probably a predisposition to uterine infection (see sections 11.8 and 11.9).
- Reduction in the speed of uterine involution (see section 5.5).
- Reduction in the first-service and subsequent pregnancy rates and extension of the calving-to-conception interval (see section 7.10).
- Increased probability of being culled.

The average total cost in 1995 in the UK for each case of placental retention was £289 which includes a figure of £6–25 for the direct cost of treatment.

10.5   TREATMENT

Opinions vary on the value of different treatment regimens because of problems of accurately quantifying the response. Herdsmen dislike working with cows with placental retention, especially in the milking parlour, because of the unpleasant odour; therefore pressure is exerted for its rapid manual removal. Considerable trauma can be caused to the uterus if manual removal is attempted before the placenta will readily detach. The following regimen should be considered:

- The herdsman should be advised to cut off those portions of the placenta that are hanging from the vulva.
- Manual removal should not be attempted if the cow is ill and has pyrexia. Systemic broad spectrum antibiotics should be given.
- Manual removal should not be attempted before 4 days postpartum and then it should consist of gentle but steady traction on the placental mass

contained within the vagina. The hand should not be forced through the cervix.

- Intra-uterine therapy is of little value. A therapeutic dose of a broad spectrum antibiotic is preferable but requires the withholding of milk for consumption.
- Oxytocin, prostaglandin $F_2\alpha$ or analogues and other hormones are of little or no value.
- All cows that have had placental retention should be examined at about 3–4 weeks postpartum to assess the degree of uterine involution and the absence of uterine infection (see sections 5.5 and 11.9).

11 Problems During the Puerperium

11.1 INTRODUCTION

The normal puerperium is considered in Chapter 5. Problems during this phase of the cow's reproductive life can have profound effects, causing infertility and sterility (Chapter 7). Many of the problems can be prevented by good obstetrical practice (Chapter 9).

11.2 LACERATIONS OF THE VULVA AND VAGINA

These occur most frequently following dystocia and are associated with rough obstetrical manipulations; they rarely if ever occur in the absence of such interference.

Vaginal lacerations

These occur when severe traction has been used, especially if there is inadequate lubrication, when the vagina is not relaxed and where there is a slight stricture, and when attempts at extension of the limbs are made without adequate repulsion.

The cow will show signs of pelvic discomfort with frequent straining and voiding of fluid exudate and perhaps debris (including retro-peritoneal fat in old, fat cows). The lesions often become infected with opportunist pathogens, particularly *Fusobacterium necrophorum*.

Treat with caudal epidural anaesthesia using a local anaesthetic solution and xylazine, to give temporary relief and perhaps break the straining cycle, and with systemic antibiotics and local emollient creams.

Vulval lacerations

These frequently involve the perineum in general. They arise where there is feto-maternal disproportion, where there is vulval stricture or stenosis (see section 9.8) or where excessive traction, particularly with the indiscriminate use of a calving aid (see section 9.7), is applied before the vulva has relaxed and become capable of being stretched.

Superficial lacerations of the first-degree involve mucosa and skin and should be sutured as soon as possible after they occur.

Second-degree lacerations involve deeper tissues such as the constrictor muscles of the vulva and should also be sutured immediately. Healing without repair can lead to pneumovagina and infertility.

Third-degree lacerations involve the vulva, vaginal wall, anal sphincter and rectum so that a cloaca is formed (see Fig. 11.1). Treatment should be delayed for about 6 weeks until cicatrization occurs, after which the Aanes' method should be used. Failure to repair will lead to faecal contamination of the vagina, pneumovagina, vaginitis and metritis.

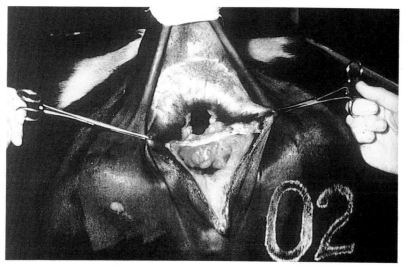

Fig. 11.1 Cow with third-degree perineal laceration. Note that the breakdown of tissue between rectum and vestibule/vagina creates a cloaca.

Vulval lacerations can be prevented by the technique of episiotomy (see Fig. 11.2) and carefully controlled traction.

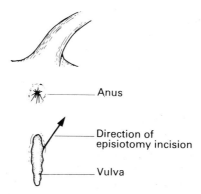

Fig. 11.2. Site of episiotomy incision.

11.3   CONTUSIONS OF THE GENITAL TRACT

These are very common as a result of feto-maternal disproportion or traction without adequate lubrication. Mild contusions are of little consequence, but excessive ones might be associated with damage to deeper tissues (see section 11.5).

11.4   HAEMATOMAS

These are usually associated with rough obstetrical practice although they can occur following normal birth. If they are large and are present before expulsion of the calf they can cause obstruction and dystocia, in which case aseptic drainage using a hypodermic needle is required. If present after the birth of the calf they should not be drained. Abscesses sometimes occur as a consequence.

11.5   PERIPHERAL NERVE DAMAGE

Severe contusions of the vagina are often associated with damage to the peripheral nerves in the pelvis by pressure from the skeleton of the calf during traction. Nerve damage can be unilateral or bilateral.

- *Obturator nerve paralysis.* The obturator nerve innervates the muscles of adduction of the hind limbs. If paralysis is bilateral, the cow may find difficulty in rising when recumbent. When standing and walking the limb(s) are abducted and there is a danger of the cow 'doing the splits' and fracturing the neck of the femur, rupturing the round ligament or dislocating the hip.

  Treatment involves good nursing, plenty of deep bedding (muck and straw) and hobbling the hind limbs to prevent over-abduction. Time will usually result in a cure.
- *Gluteal nerve paralysis.* The gluteal nerve innervates the muscles surrounding the pelvis and hind limbs. The cow will find great difficulty in rising when recumbent and supporting its full weight.

  Treatment involves good nursing, as described above. Regular attempts to lift the cow with a pneumatic bed or 'Bagshaw' hoist prevent other injuries and cramp.

11.6   UTERINE TEARS

These can occur during normal calving or dystocia where there is manipulation; there may be considerable haemorrhage from the vulva.

Suturing is rarely feasible and, since involution will reduce the size of the tear (see section 5.5), oxytocin can be injected to hasten the process.

The prognosis will depend upon the site of the tear and whether the calf was alive or dead and putrefying. If the tear is dorsal and the calf was alive then the prognosis is good. If the tear is ventral and the calf putrefying, the prognosis is bad and the cow should be slaughtered.

Uterine tears can have a long-term effect upon fertility and may cause sterility.

11.7 UTERINE PROLAPSE

The colloquial term is 'casting the calf-bed'. Prolapse occurs following about 0.5% of calvings.

Most occur within 4–6 h of calving, although occasionally up to 36–48 h. The cow is frequently recumbent and may have had dystocia which has been relieved by traction. There is rarely any problem in identifying the condition although it has been mistaken for retained placenta.

Predisposing factors:

- The age of the cow. Prolapse is most common in old dairy cows.
- Hypocalcaemia – with or without clinical signs of milk fever and recumbency.
- Dystocia — especially following traction in beef heifers.
- Prepartum vaginal prolapse (see section 8.12) – there is some association with this condition.
- Placental retention (see sections 10.1–10.4).

How does the uterus prolapse? This is not accurately known, but it is possible to speculate:

- The tip of the horn of the flaccid uterus, perhaps with the placenta still attached, becomes invaginated.
- This stimulates uterine contractions, which exacerbate the invagination.
- Once this reaches the pelvis it stimulates straining and the uterus is completely everted.

Treatment. Immediately the prolapse is identified the herdsman can do much to help the condition:

- Remove other cows, or isolate the cow with the prolapse, to prevent trauma induced by other cows sniffing and trampling on the organ.
- Cover the organ with wet towels or sheets and if possible support it above the level of the vagina to prevent or reduce passive venous congestion.
- On arrival at the farm, quickly check the general health of the cow, especially the pulse and mucous membranes for evidence of haemorrhage. If she is severely hypocalcaemic treat with calcium borogluconate; if it is a mild case leave untreated until the prolapse has been replaced.

- If the cow is recumbent place her on her sternum with both hind legs extended backwards. Give caudal epidural anaesthesia.
- If the cow is standing, support the uterus above the level of the vulva, with the help of two assistants, with a towel or sheet on either side.
- Clean the uterus thoroughly with saline or warm water (no disinfectant).
- Check for evidence of tears. If any are present suture with absorbable sutures (chromic catgut).
- Attempt to remove the placenta if it is still attached and readily separates from the caruncles; if not, cut off the dependent portions and leave attached.
- Firmly but gently, using the palms of the hand or fist, start to replace the prolapsed organ starting at the part adjacent to the vulva (see Fig. 11.3). The procedure becomes more difficult as more of the prolapsed organ is replaced. The last portion is the most difficult and frequently requires an assistant to pull open the vulva.
- Once the organ has passed through the vulva it must be pushed cranially and ventrally to ensure that the prolapse is completely reduced and the uterus returned to normal. This is aided by using the fist and arm in a pumping action; the length of the arm can be extended by grasping a wine bottle and inserting that as a plunger. Alternatively, several litres of physiological saline can be infused to evert the organ, which can subsequently be siphoned off.
- Inject calcium borogluconate, 50 iu of oxytocin and systemic broad spectrum antibiotics.
- Close the vulva with two mattress sutures of nylon tape inserted in the perivulval tissue.
- Re-examine the cow in 12–24 h, remove the vulval sutures and palpate the vagina to ensure that the uterus has not re-prolapsed and that the cervix has partially constricted.

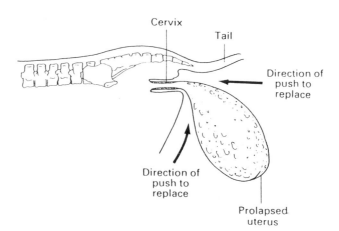

Fig. 11.3. Method of replacement of prolapsed uterus.

- If the prolapse cannot be replaced then amputation is an extreme method of treatment or preferably the cow should be slaughtered.

Prognosis. The ease of replacement and the prognosis will depend upon the duration that the organ has been prolapsed, together with the amount of trauma and the ability to remove the placenta readily. All cows will develop metritis of varying severity (see section 11.8).

The calving-to-conception interval will be extended; some cows will be rendered sterile.

11.8   ACUTE METRITIS

This occurs at varying periods postpartum, although most cases will be within 7 days of calving.

There is a *history* of dystocia treated by manipulation and/or traction with the removal of a dead, often putrefying, calf, or placental retention, or uterine prolapse. The cow has become ill, with loss of appetite, reduced milk yield, lethargy and dullness. She may strain periodically, especially if there is a concurrent vaginitis, and there may be a sero-sanguinous, evil-smelling discharge.

Clinical examination will show pyrexia and raised pulse and respiration rates. Mastitis and pneumonia must be eliminated. Vaginal examination should not be made in the acute phase; a rectal examination will allow palpation of the uterus which will be poorly involuted.

Treatment. Give caudal epidural anaesthesia to stop the cow straining (see section 11.2). Broad spectrum systemic antibiotics, supportive fluid therapy and good nursing are also required.

Prognosis is guarded – some cows will become toxaemic and die, others will show an improvement in general health within 24 h. If the latter, vaginal examination can be done and the uterus lavaged with 5–10 l of physiological saline which is quickly siphoned off. Inevitably most cases of metritis develop into chronic endometritis (see section 11.9 below).

11.9   CHRONIC ENDOMETRITIS

Strictly speaking, this implies inflammation of the endometrium. However, it is difficult to know if the deeper layers of the uterine wall are also involved.

History. Chronic endometritis is usually found in isolated individual cows (some of which will have had acute metritis and recovered) with a muco-purulent vulval discharge (leucorrhoea or 'whites') several weeks after calving. The majority will have had no obvious post-partum complications other than, perhaps, placental retention, but will show leucorrhoea. On some farms considerable numbers of cows may be affected in some years.

Clinical examination. The cow will show no signs of ill health; appetite and milk yield will be normal. Vaginal examination will show the presence of varying quantities of mucopurulent material of varying consistency, ranging from thick pus to thin mucus containing flecks of purulent material. Rectal palpation will demonstrate that in most cases the uterus is slightly larger than it should be (poorly involuted) and will have an oedematous or 'doughy' feel; in some cases it may be distended with pus (pyometra – see section 11.10). The ovaries may or may not show signs of cyclical activity (see section 1.14 and Table 1.1).

Causes. In some cases the condition may be a sequel to an acute metritis. Most cases arise because of the failure to eliminate the uterine bacterial contamination that occurs in most cows postpartum (see sections 5.7 and 5.8). This failure may be due to the following:

- Excessive bacterial contamination overwhelming natural defence mechanisms.
- Placental retention.
- Poor uterine involution.
- Deficient defence mechanisms – macrophage activity and the immune system.
- Delayed return or, perhaps, premature return to oestrus after calving.
- Tissue injury.
- Nature of bacterial flora – notably the role of *Actinomyces pyogenes* and gram-negative anaerobes, especially those of the bacteroides species.

Treatment. There has been little meaningful evaluation of different treatments. The following are the methods used:

- If a CL is palpable on one of the ovaries, prostaglandin $F_{2\alpha}$ or analogue will lyse the CL, hasten the return to oestrus and shorten the luteal phase. Both these procedures increase the ability of the genital tract to eliminate infection.
- If there is no CL palpable, an intramuscular injection of 3 mg oestradiol benzoate is indicated.
- Intra-uterine infusion of a *therapeutic dose* of a broad spectrum antibiotic such as oxytetracyclines; milk must be withdrawn from use.
- Intramuscular injection of a broad spectrum antibiotic such as oxytetracyclines; milk must be withdrawn from use.

Effect upon fertility. Endometritis will depress fertility by extending the calving-to-conception interval (see section 7.10). Some cows may become sterile because of irreversible changes in the tubular genital tract. It is unlikely that endometritis in the absence of clinical signs will have much effect upon fertility (see section 7.7).

11.10 PYOMETRA

This implies the accumulation of pus in the uterus.

History. There is no observed oestrus (see section 7.6), and perhaps a history of intermittent leucorrhoea.

Clinical examination may show some evidence of mucopurulent material in the vagina. Rectal palpation will show an enlarged uterus, which should be *differentiated from pregnancy* (see section 2.11 and Fig. 7.2), and a CL on one ovary.

Treatment. Prostaglandin $F_2\alpha$ or analogue will lyse the CL and the cow will come into oestrus and eliminate the infection.

12 Manipulation of Reproduction

12.1 TWINNING AND MULTIPLE OVULATIONS

Normally, after oestrus, a single follicle ovulates and only one oocyte is shed. The incidence of twinning is about 1–2% and of triplets 0.013%.

Increasing the plane of nutrition by flushing does not increase the ovulation rate. This can only be achieved by:

- genetic selection, which is not very successful.
- use of exogenous gonadotrophic hormones. The response is unpredictable.

Embryo transfer techniques can be used to produce twins (see below).

Desirability of inducing twinning
Problems can occur as a result of twin calves:

- High incidence of retained placenta (see section 10.2).
- Dystocia with high calf mortality (see section 9.8).
- Reduced milk yield.
- Subsequent reduced fertility of the dam.
- Freemartin calves.

Some of these problems can be overcome if it is known that a cow is carrying twins, so that additional feeding can be given and greater attention can be paid at the time of calving.

12.2 EMBRYO TRANSFER

This is the technique by which embryos are collected from the genital tract of one cow (the donor) and are transferred to the genital tract of another cow (the recipient), in which gestation is completed.

Applications of embryo transfer
When combined with superovulation of the donor the applications are as follows:

- The increase in the number of offspring from genetically superior cows.
- The increase in the speed of progeny testing.
- The reduction of the generation interval by superovulating prepubertal heifers and transferral of the embryos to mature recipients. This can increase the speed of genetic selection.
- The transportation of embryos from country to country so as to overcome problems of disease spread and the need for quarantine. The possible danger of diseases – especially viral – being spread must be considered and the necessary precautions taken.
- Induction of twinning.
- Embryos can be obtained from infertile cows that may not be capable of sustaining normal pregnancy.
- Embryo transfer can be used as a research tool.

Requirements for successful embryo transfer

A source of embryos from a suitable donor. Although a single embryo can be collected and transferred, more embryos can be collected and transferred when superovulation is induced.

- A sufficient number of recipients, whose oestrous cycles are synchronised with that of the donor, to receive the harvested embryos.
- The availability of equipment for cryopreservation of embryos.

Conduct of embryo transfer

In the UK, embryo transfer in cattle is governed by statute under the Bovine Embryo (Collection, Production and Transfer) Regulations 1995 and the Veterinary Surgery (Epidural Anaesthesia) Order 1992. This legislation provides a framework so that embryo transfer can be performed effectively, efficiently and, more importantly, without detriment to the health and welfare of donors and recipients. Veterinarians involved in embryo transfer must be familiar with the legislation, competent and sufficiently experienced if they are leading a collection team.

Selection of the donor

- She will have been chosen by the owner because she is of high genetic merit or she may be infertile.
- It must be at least 2 months since she last calved.
- She must have normal reproductive structure and function.

Selection of recipients

- Heifers or young cows.
- They must have normal reproductive structure and function.
- They must have calved at least 2 months ago.
- *They must be of adequate size and maturity so that, knowing the breed and type of embryo to be implanted, they will be capable of carrying the calf to term and calve naturally.*

Superovulatory hormones

A number of different supervulatory gonadotrophins have been, and are, used in embryo transfer.

- Equine chorionic gonadotrophin (eCG) is inexpensive, but it has a longer biological half-life than bovine FSH, producing an exaggerated response with poor recovery of embryos and aberrant ovarian activity for some time afterwards. Better results are obtained when used in conjunction with eCG antiserum.
- Human menopausal gonadotrophin (hMG).
- Porcine pituitary preparations; those preparations that have been purified so that they have consistent FSH but low LH concentrations.
- Ovine pituitary preparations.
- Equine pituitary preparations.
- Recombinant bovine FSH (bFSH).

Preparation and superovulation of the donor

(see Fig. 12.1)
There are many variations in the regimens that are used to induce super-ovulation of the donor cow. This will depend upon the superovulatory

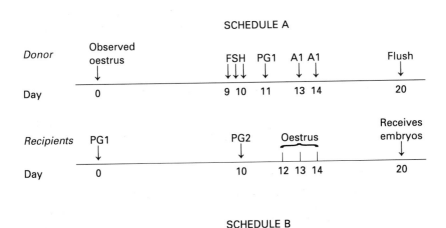

Fig. 12.1. Donor and recipient treatment regimens for embryo transfer.

preparation used, for example, eCG requires a single injection whereas hMG or pituitary-derived FSH preparations require repeated injections. In addition, individuals involved in embryo transfer have their own regimens arrived at from previous experience. However, it is important that protocols are followed precisely.

- The donor is either observed for the signs of oestrus and the date recorded (Schedule A), or given two injections of prostaglandin $F_{2\alpha}$ ($PGF_{2\alpha}$) 11 days apart (PG1 and PG2) (Schedule B). It is assumed that oestrus will occur 2–3 days after PG2 (see Fig. 12.1); it should be detected and recorded.
- A superovulatory dose of porcine FSH is injected on three separate days, 9–13 days after observed oestrus (Schedule A) or 12–16 days after PG2 (Schedule B). If eCG is used, a single injection only is given.
- Forty-eight hours after the first FSH (or single eCG) injection, PG1 (Schedule A) or PG3 (Schedule B) should be given. The donor should be in oestrus 2 days later; it should be observed and recorded.
- The donor should be inseminated during oestrus with a repeat 12 h later. There are several variations on these regimens particularly regarding the number and timing of AI.
- Embryos are flushed 7–8 days after the first AI.
- If the donor does not return to oestrus 28 days after flushing she should be treated with $PGF_{2\alpha}$ to prevent the possibility of pregnancy with multiple embryos.

Preparation of recipients

For the best results the oestrous cycles of recipients should be accurately synchronised with that of the donor; more than 1 day of asynchrony will reduce the pregnancy rates. At least twelve recipients per donor should be available if provision for freezing embryos is not available.

Two schedules are possible:

- If Schedule A is used for the donor (Fig. 12.1) then the recipients are injected with PG1 on day 0 with PG2 10 days later.
- If Schedule B is used for the donor then each recipient has PG1 on day 2, PG2 on day 13 and PG3 on day 24 (16–24h before the donor receives PG3); the luteolytic response is more rapid in the donor after FSH or eCG priming.
- Oestrus should be observed on days 12, 13 and 14 (Schedule A) or 26, 27 and 28 (Schedule B) and recorded. Recipients receive embryos on day 20 (Schedule A) or 34 (Schedule B).
- Other methods of synchronisation can be used, such as progesterone-intravaginal devices (PRID and CIDR, see section 1.12) together with $PGF_{2\alpha}$ either before or at the time of withdrawal.

Collection of embryos

Initially embryos were recovered surgically under general anaesthesia via a mid-line laparotomy. This technique has been superseded by non-surgical methods. The embryos are collected on day 6 or day 7 when they are late morulas or early blastocysts (see section 2.3):

- The donor is suitably restrained in a crush or stocks.
- Caudal epidural anaesthesia is induced. Sedation may be necessary: spasmolytic drugs and β_2 mimetics can be used.
- The rectum is evacuated of faeces.
- The vulva and perineum are thoroughly cleansed and the whole procedure performed as aseptically as possible.
- There are basically two methods of flushing embryos from the uterine horns of superovulated donors. One method uses a three-way fixed distance Foley PVC catheter (see Fig. 12.2), the other uses a two-way Foley rubber catheter (see Fig. 12.3).
- The three-way catheter is inserted into the uterine horns using a speculum and cervical dilator with introducer (see Figs. 12.4 and 12.5). The two-way catheter is inserted using a tightly fitting stilet or stiffener and a conventional AI technique.
- The cuff is inflated to occlude the lumen of the horn.
- 300 ml of flushing medium (enriched phosphate-buffered saline, EPS) warmed to body temperature is infused using a syringe in 50 ml aliquots. The flushings are collected in 50–100 ml aliquots; the horn is gently squeezed *per rectum* to displace embryos.
- When most of the flushing medium has been collected, the cuff is deflated and the catheter removed. A second, sterile Foley catheter is now inserted into the opposite horn and the procedure repeated.

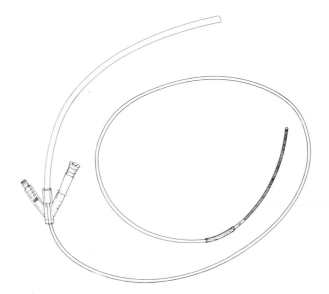

Fig. 12.2. Three-way Foley PVC catheter.

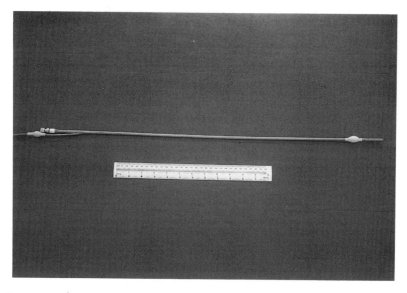

Fig. 12.3. Two-way Foley rubber catheter with stilet inserted for recovery of embryos.

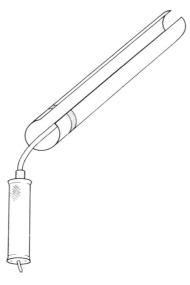

Fig. 12.4. Speculum with incomplete cylinder, used to insert cervical cannula.

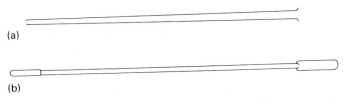

(a)

(b)

Fig. 12.5. Cervical cannula (a), and trochar (b), used for non-surgical recovery of embryos using a three-way Foley catheter.

Recovery of the embryos

- The collecting vessels (boiling tubes or graduated cylinders) are allowed to stand for 30 min. The majority of the fluid is decanted so that 20–30ml remains. This is then searched using a round-bottomed collection dish and a microscope at a low magnification.
- Each embryo is carefully aspirated into a Pasteur pipette and transferred into fresh EPS for evaluation.
- The embryos will be at slightly different stages of development. Evaluation is done on morphological appearance and requires expert assessment. A qualitative assessment is given as a measure of its likelihood of developing into a normal calf.
- Embryos remain viable for about 7 h in EPS medium. They can be cultured for 12 h in fetal calf serum if there is any doubt about their normality, and then re-examined.

Transfer of the embryos

Two methods are used, either surgical or non-surgical. The latter technique has been superseded by the former in the interest of the welfare of recipients.

- *Surgical transfer.* This is preferably done via a high left sub-lumbar fossa laparotomy under paravertebral anaesthesia using normal aseptic techniques. The embryo is aspirated into a Pasteur pipette with 0.5 ml of EPS and is deposited with the medium into the uterine horn adjacent to the CL. A blunt 16 G needle is used to make a small puncture in the wall of the uterine horn.
- *Non-surgical transfer.* This is done using a slightly modified Cassou AI

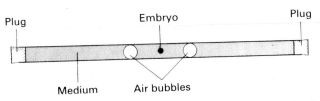

Fig. 12.6. Diagram to show the method of placing the embryo in the AI straw before non-surgical transfer.

pipette (see section 14.4). Each embryo, together with a small volume of EPS, is aspirated into a conventional semen straw (see section 14.3) with a small bubble of air on either side to aid identification (see Fig. 12.6). The ovaries are gently palpated to assess which ovary contains the CL.

The straw is placed in the Cassou pipette. The cow is restrained in a crush, under caudal epidural anaesthesia. The vulva and perineum are very thoroughly cleaned. The pipette is inserted into the external os of the cervix, and gently introduced using a normal AI procedure (see section 14.4). It is carefully advanced along the horn adjacent to the CL and the plunger firmly depressed to expel the embryo. The pipette is carefully withdrawn.

Palpation of the genital tract should be as minimal as possible and the technique must be performed with strict attention to cleanliness. The quality of the CL of the recipient is frequently assessed qualitatively by rectal palpation or ultrasonography and also by measuring peripheral progesterone concentrations.

12.3   FREEZING AND STORAGE OF EMBRYOS

Embryos can be successfully stored in liquid nitrogen using glycerol as a cryoprotectant. Recent work has shown ethylene glycol to be effective. Plastic 0.25 and 0.5 ml straws are normally used for freezing and storage. Pregnancy rates are not as good as those following the use of fresh embryos.

12.4   MICROMANIPULATION OF EMBRYOS

Monozygotic twins have been produced by dividing the morulas or early blastocysts flushed from a donor. This is done by micromanipulation under a microscope and successful pregnancies have been obtained by transferring the divided blastocysts to synchronised recipients.

12.5   *IN VITRO* MATURATION AND FERTILISATION OF OOCYTES

Immature oocytes aspirated from 2–5 mm diameter follicles in ovaries recovered from abattoirs have been used as a source of cheap embryos. More recently, in genetically superior cows, oocytes have been recovered by aspiration using guidance with transvaginal ultrasound imaging; up to an average of nine oocytes have been recovered on each occasion even when aspirations were performed frequently.

Recovered oocytes are cultured for about 24 h in a medium containing serum from oestrous cows. When mature, they are cultured with capacitated sperm. Fertilised oocytes are then further cultured until they reach morala or early blastocyst stages before they are frozen or transferred to recipients.

Part 2
The Male

13   Normal Male Animal

13.1   REPRODUCTIVE ANATOMY OF THE BULL

The three main components of the reproductive system are:

- the testes;
- the accessory sex organs, namely the epididymides, ductus deferens, vesicular glands (seminal vesicles), prostate and bulbo-urethral glands;
- the penis.

They are represented diagramatically in Fig. 13.1.

The testes – structure and function

The testes descend from the abdomen about midway through fetal life. In the mature bull they are about $13 \times 7 \times 7$ cm and oval in shape, weigh about 350 g and are more or less equal in size. The testes are enclosed within a tough connective tissue capsule, the tunica albuginea, which retains the testicular tissue under tension. This gives the testes their characteristic texture on palpation, i.e. slightly fluctuating.

The testis comprises a mass of convoluted seminiferous tubules in which sperm production occurs (spermatogenesis), and interstitial tissue containing the Leydig cells. The seminiferous tubules comprise a basement membrane, germ cells that give rise to spermatozoa and Sertoli cells which have many functions, namely they secrete tubule fluids, pyruvate, lactate, inhibin, oestrogens, and proteins (see Fig. 13.2). Cell division occurs and the various types of germ cell progress from the spermatogonia, adjacent to the basement membrane, through the primary and secondary spermatocytes and spermatids to spermatozoa, which are present in the central lumen of the tubules (see Fig. 13.2). During this process of spermatogenesis, which takes about 54 days in the bull, the number of chromosomes is reduced to half the normal number (haploid).

The Leydig cells appear to have an endocrine function only, producing testosterone.

Endocrine function

FSH regulates spermatogenesis mainly by its effects upon the Sertoli cells

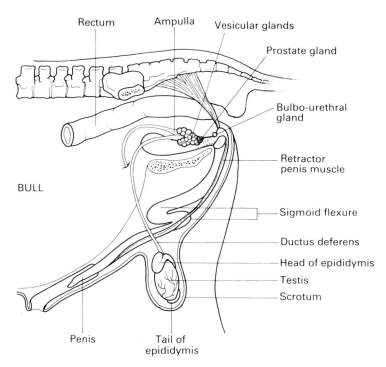

Fig. 13.1. Diagram of the genital system of the bull. (Reproduced from Ashdown, R. & Hancock, J.L. (1980) *Reproduction in Farm Animals*, 4th edn, (ed. E.S.E. Hafez). Lea & Febiger, Philadelphia.)

where it stimulates the secretion of pyruvate and lactate, both of which are thought necessary as energy sources for the germinal epithelial cells, and androgen binding protein (ABP). This latter substance ensures the maintenance of high concentrations of androgens in the seminiferous and epididymal tubules. FSH also stimulates the Sertoli cells to convert testosterone to oestrogens.

LH stimulates the secretion of testosterone from the Leydig cells as well as playing an important role in the control of spermatogenesis; testosterone is also responsible for libido, secondary sex characteristics and accessory gland function.

Secretion of FSH is regulated by the negative feedback effect of reproductive steroid hormones and inhibin, LH by testosterone.

Epididymis

This is a convoluted tube of about 30 m in length, closely attached to the surface of each testis, and comprising a head, body and tail (see Fig. 13.1). Spermatozoa are transported along the seminiferous tubes as a suspension in fluid, through the rete testis and efferent ducts to the head of the epididymis. Sperm in the heads of the epididymides are immotile and

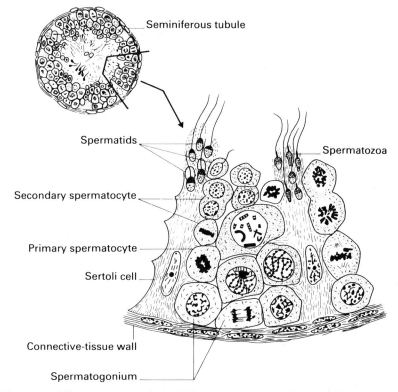

Seminiferous tubule

Spermatids

Spermatozoa

Secondary spermatocyte

Primary spermatocyte

Sertoli cell

Connective-tissue wall

Spermatogonium

Fig. 13.2. Microstructure of seminiferous tubules to show cell layers. (Reproduced from Hunter, R.F.H. (1980) *Reproduction in Farm Animals*, 4th edn (ed. E.S.E. Hafez). Lea & Febiger, Philadelphia.)

incapable of fertilising; however, as they proceed distally towards the tail the ability of both functions develops although is not exhibited until ejaculated. They reside there for about 11–8 days. In the epididymis there is:

- concentration of spermatozoa;
- maturation of spermatozoa;
- storage of spermatozoa.

Ductus deferens and ampulla

These enable spermatozoa to pass from the tail of the epididymis to the urethra; the ampullae also act as stores.

Prostate gland

This is a collar-like structure which produces accessory fluid. Rarely is it a site of disease in the bull.

Vesicular glands (seminal vesicles)

These are paired, compact, lobulated, flask-shaped glands about 12 cm in length, 5 cm wide and 3 cm thick, situated in the pelvis adjacent to the urethra (see Fig. 13.1); they produce accessory fluid rich in fructose. They can be a site of infection (see section 15.8).

Bulbo-urethral glands

These are paired glands that are not palpable, and are reputed to be the source of the precopulatory preputial secretion (see section 13.3).

The penis

The bull has a fibro-elastic type of penis with a sigmoid flexure. Erection mainly involves the obliteration of the flexure so that the penis is straight; there is only a slight increase in length.

Erection occurs due to engorgement of the two corpora cavernosa penis (CCP) and to a lesser extent the corpus spongiosum penis (CSP) (see Fig. 13.3) with blood. Initially there is increased arterial blood supply to the CCP followed by rhythmical contractions of the ischiocavernosus muscles which helps to pump blood into the distal closed spaces of the CCP and at the same time occludes the venous drainage from the CCP. There is a massive increase in pressure in the CCP to 100 × normal arterial pressure, which straightens the sigmoid flexure and produces erection.

Once the ischiocavernosus muscles stop contracting, detumescence occurs and the sigmoid flexure is re-established.

13.2 PUBERTY

Puberty is the stage when the bull develops the desire to mate (libido), the ability to mate and the ability to fertilise. Young bulls frequently mount and

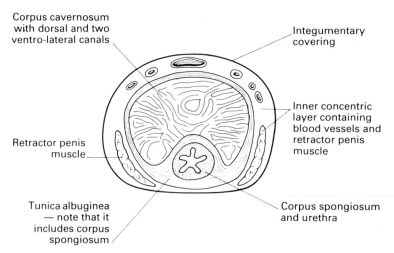

Fig. 13.3. Cross-section of bull's penis to show vascular stricture. (Reproduced from Cox, J.E. (1987) *Surgery of the Reproductive Tract of Large Animals*. Liverpool University Press, Liverpool.)

apparently show libido at several months of age, but are incapable of producing spermatozoa. Puberty develops gradually and occurs at about 9–10 months of age; it is largely dependent upon the bull reaching a certain age and weight threshold. The time of onset of puberty is influenced by:

- The breed of bull – puberty is slightly earlier in dairy breeds than in beef breeds. There is also variation within breeds.
- Body weight and growth rate and, hence, the plane of nutrition.
- Environment.

Although puberty occurs at 9–10 months of age full sexual maturity is not reached until about 2–3 years of age, depending upon the breed.

13.3   COPULATORY BEHAVIOUR

This is relatively brief, once the bull has elicited that the cow is in oestrus by licking and sniffing her vulva and then resting his chin on the rump of the cow to see if she will stand. Evidence of erection can be seen before mounting as movement in the sheath and there will usually be drops of preputial secretion (see section 13.1, bulbo-urethral glands). The bull mounts, the penis is protruded, the vulva identified and intromission achieved.

Ejaculation is always associated with a vigorous thrusting movement of the pelvis, requiring a good foothold. Failure to thrust indicates that ejaculation has not occurred. Dismounting occurs quickly and the bull may serve the cow several times in quick succession.

13.4   CLINICAL EXAMINATION OF THE BULL FOR BREEDING FITNESS

This is done at the time of purchase of a bull or where infertility in a herd or group suggests that the bull might be responsible. The procedure is as follows.

- *History*. A detailed history is required with information relating to:

1 Age of bull and origin.
2 Previous fertility, if known.
3 Time resident on present premises.
4 History of injuries or illness.
5 Method of husbandry and service procedure.
6 Number and experience of persons handling the bull.
7 Environment in which he is kept, and whether there has been any change.
8 Time interval since last service.
9 Frequency of service.
10 If a proven sire, time interval since he last sired a calf.
11 If a query about his fertility, the nature of the problem or complaint.

- *Observe service behaviour*. The behaviour in response to a cow or heifer in oestrus should be observed in the bull's *normal environment* (at least two animals should be available and in oestrus following injection with prostaglandin $F_2\alpha$ (see sections 1.11 and 1.13). From this it will be possible to assess the standard of husbandry and handling and to determine if his libido is normal or if he is unable to serve. It will also enable a visual inspection of the erect penis to be made.
- *Clinical examination*. A general clinical examination should be made with particular reference to the locomotor and genital system. The procedure for examining the genital system is as follows: (1) palpate scrotum, testes, epididymides, spermatic cords and inguinal mammary glands; measure scrotal circumference; (2) palpate sigmoid flexure, penis and prepuce; (3) assess the size of the preputial opening and look for the presence of abnormal secretions or lesions; (4) perform rectal palpation of internal genitalia, particularly palpation of the vesicular glands.
- *Semen collection*. If the bull has served the teaser cow repeatedly it is preferable to attempt semen collection after a 7-day sexual rest. The methods are described in section 13.5.

13.5   METHODS OF SEMEN COLLECTION

A number of methods can be used to collect semen:

- *Aspiration from the vagina*. If semen cannot be collected by any other method, the bull is allowed to serve naturally and some of the ejaculate can then be aspirated from the vagina. Quantitative evaluation cannot be done, but the presence of spermatozoa can be demonstrated.
- *Massage of ampullae per rectum*. This is not a very satisfactory method.
- *Electro-ejaculation*. This is a satisfactory method of collecting semen, but it can cause distress and discomfort and should not be used unless the person responsible for the procedure is experienced and has the appropriate equipment. It should not be used for repeated collection.
- *Artificial vagina*. This is the most satisfactory method of collection. Provided that a teaser cow in oestrus is available, most bulls will mount and serve into an artificial vagina (AV).

  Essentially this comprises a rigid rubber cylinder into which is inserted a latex rubber liner so that a water jacket can be created (see Figs 13.4 and 13.5). A latex rubber cone with collecting vessel is attached. Water at between 42°C and 46°C is used in the water jacket and the inner surface of the latex liner is covered with a thin smear of obstetrical jelly. The bull is allowed to mount and the penis is deflected, by holding it through the prepuce, into the AV. Immediately the bull should thrust vigorously, ejaculate and, as the bull dismounts, the semen will be seen

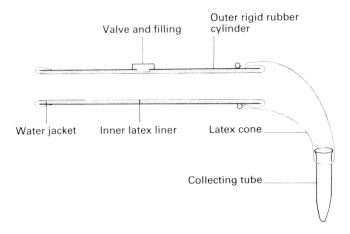

Fig. 13.4. Diagram of an artificial vagina.

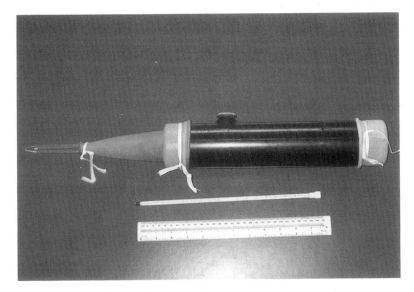

Fig. 13.5. An artificial vagina assembled for semen collection.

to have been deposited in the tube; it should be immediately protected from temperature shock and u.v. light.

13.6 SEMEN COMPOSITION

- Volume: 6 ml (range 2–12 ml).
- Colour: creamy yellow to milky white.
- Sperm concentration: 1200 (range 500–2500) $\times$ 10^6 per ml.
- Sperm output per ejaculate: 7500 (range 2000–15 000) $\times$ 10^6.

13.7   SEMEN EVALUATION

The following evaluation can be performed with modest equipment:

- Volume: this can be recorded immediately if a graduated tube is used.
- Colour: this can be assessed and recorded immediately. The presence of blood-staining, faeces, urine or pus contamination should be noted to enable further clinical examination to be done.
- Mass motility: this should be assessed immediately on the farm. A heated stage or heated surface should be available. A drop of semen placed on a slide is examined under low power for signs of vigorous wave motion; this is assessed subjectively and given a score between 5 and 0.
- Individual motility of sperm: this can be assessed using a warmed diluted sample of semen (physiological saline) under a high power of magnification.
- Number of live sperm: this can be assessed using a stained smear. This is made of diluted semen with a vital stain such as nigrosin-eosin. Dead or moribund sperm are stained pink; live sperm do not stain and appear white against the deep blue background. The percentage dead are counted; ideally it should be <15%.
- The morphological structure of individual spermatozoa: this can be assessed using the nigrosin-eosin-stained smear. Abnormal spermatoza should be noted, and the type of abnormality recorded. Some abnormalities can be induced by the handling of semen after collection. Identification of some abnormalities and their significance to the fertility of the bull will require the opinion of an expert. Although bulls at AI centres should have very low numbers of abnormal spermatozoa, i.e. <20%, because of the small sperm doses used compared with natural service (see section 14.4), many fertile bulls used for natural service have greater numbers of abnormal spermatozoa. Large percentages, however, should be viewed with caution.
- The sperm concentration can be assessed approximately by noting the colour and density of the ejaculate. It is best determined using a counting chamber such as a Neubauer haemocytometer together with a red blood cell pipette to dilute the sample.

13.8   FREQUENCY OF NATURAL SERVICE

Young bulls less than two years of age should be used less frequently than mature bulls: for the former about two to four services per week; for the latter up to twelve services per week, provided this is not every week. Young bulls should not be running with more than about ten to fifteen cows or heifers; older bulls can run with up to about twenty-five. A young bull may well be bullied by cows or heifers, especially if he is not very dominant.

14   Artificial Insemination

14.1   INTRODUCTION

Artificial insemination (AI) is used extensively in many parts of the world, particularly in dairy cattle; its use in beef breeds is more restricted because of the problems of oestrus detection (see section 1.8) and handling, although, with the development of effective oestrus synchronisation methods, many of these problems have been overcome (see sections 1.10–1.13).

Advantages

- Extensive use can be made of superior sires.
- Semen can be stored, when frozen, for many years after the bull is dead.
- Semen can be used from bulls after they have been progeny-tested.
- Venereal disease can be controlled, provided that there is careful screening and monitoring of bulls at AI centres.
- Farm safety is improved because potentially dangerous dairy bulls need not be kept.
- The need to rear and feed a bull on the farm is removed.

Disadvantages

- Oestrus needs to be detected and insemination timed accurately (see sections 1.8 and 14.4) in order to obtain good pregnancy rates.
- Dystocia can result if semen from exotic breeds is used on immature heifers.
- There is a possibility of inbreeding if there is extensive use of a limited number of sires.
- There is a possibility of extensive transfer of undesirable genetic traits if bulls are not carefully monitored.
- There is the possibility of extensive dissemination of venereal and other important infectious diseases if surveillance is inadequate at AI centres by AI personnel.

14.2 SEMEN COLLECTION

It is standard practice to use the artificial vagina (AV) for semen collection. Bulls are trained to mount teaser cows, steers or dummies. Great care is taken to prevent contamination of the ejaculate. Each bull has his own AV.

In order to increase the volume of the ejaculate and the number of spermatozoa ejaculated, bulls are usually teased before collection. The collection procedure is described in section 13.5.

14.3 HANDLING AND PROCESSING OF SEMEN – GENERAL PRINCIPLES

Fresh raw semen can be used, although there is a danger of the spread of disease; its use is prohibited in the UK.

Practically all AI involves the use of frozen semen. Freezing has distinct advantages in that semen can be stored for a long time even after the bull has died; it enables the ready transport of semen worldwide; and, provided that there is careful quarantine and handling, it prevents the spread of disease. Semen has to be protected from the effects of freezing and handling which would result in the death of spermatozoa. For this reason a diluent or extender is added to the semen. The diluent must have the following constituents:

- A nutrient substrate, usually a sugar.
- A substance to protect the spermatozoa from damage from freezing and other temperature changes.
- A buffer to prevent changes in pH and also osmotic pressure.
- Antibiotics to kill bacteria that might be transmitted from the bull and those that might affect the spermatozoa.

A diluent also increases the number of possible doses of semen since the bull produces more spermatozoa than are necessary for fertilisation in one ejaculate.

Processing procedure

Immediately after collection the ejaculate is quickly assessed for suitability for processing. The diluents used are egg yolk citrate or more commonly heated skimmed milk with egg yolk, fructose and glycerol (the glycerol enables semen to be deep-frozen).

After the addition of diluent, the semen is placed in polyvinyl chloride straws with a capacity of between 0.25 and 0.5 ml. These straws are colour-coded to aid in identification and sealed with a polyvinyl alcohol powder plug which can also be coloured to assist in identification of the source of the semen. Details of the bull and the collection date are displayed on the side. Most straws used commercially now contain 0.25 ml of diluted semen.

The filled straws are then bundled together and cooled in the vapour above liquid nitrogen before they are plunged into the liquid nitrogen at a temperature of $-196°C$. Provided careful attention is paid to maintenance of the level of liquid nitrogen in the storage vessel, semen can be stored for years at this temperature with only minimal loss of fertilising capacity. Semen straws can also be transported in a small liquid nitrogen flask with a capacity as small as 3 l.

Once the straw has been thawed it cannot be refrozen without severely affecting the fertilising capacity of the spermatozoa; therefore straws should only be briefly removed from the liquid nitrogen flask for selection and only removed just before insemination.

Thawing before insemination

The semen in the straw must be thawed after its removal from the liquid nitrogen before insemination. This is best done by steadily increasing the temperature from that of liquid nitrogen $(-196°C)$ to that of ambient temperature or $37°C$ before it is deposited in the cow. Placing the straw in a beaker of water at $37°C$ for 7–15 s – depending on the capacity of the straw – is adequate.

14.4 INSEMINATION TECHNIQUE

The straw is removed from the glass beaker, dried with a clean tissue and the tip of one end of the straw cut off with clean scissors to remove the plug. It is then placed in the Cassou insemination pipette or gun (see Fig. 14.1).

The procedure for depositing the semen into the cow is as follows:

- The cow or heifer is adequately restrained, preferably in a crush or stall to prevent forward, backward and side-to-side movement; an assistant to hold the tail is advantageous.
- The Cassou pipette is gently held in the inseminator's teeth and if the inseminator is right-handed the left hand is inserted into the rectum to locate the cervix. If large amounts of faeces are present in the rectum defecation should be stimulated or the faeces removed.
- The vulva is thoroughly cleaned with a dry paper towel.
- The forearm is gently pressed downwards to slightly compress the vulva, which is thus partially dilated.
- The pipette is gently inserted at an angle of about 45°, with its tip directed cranially and dorsally, into the vulva and along the vaginal wall. Sometimes remnants of the hymen can impede its progress; extending the cervix cranially often helps.
- Once the tip is located in the fornix of the vagina, the cervix is grasped firmly by the left hand and the external os located with the tip of the pipette; this can usually be determined by the presence of a 'grating' sensation.

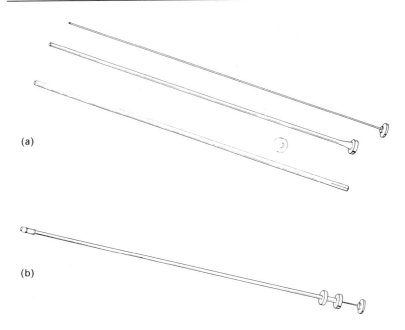

(a)

(b)

Fig. 14.1. Cassou insemination pipette, (a) dismantled and (b) assembled.

- Once the external os is located the cervix can be retracted, and using a combination of pushing the pipette through the cervical canal, and pulling the cervix onto the pipette, it should be possible to negotiate its passage. Sometimes the tip impinges upon a cervical fold, in which case the pipette should be slightly withdrawn and then redirected. The technique is easier in parous animals than in heifers and when the animal is truly in oestrus. Gentleness to prevent trauma must be the rule.
- The tip of the pipette should be sited just within the uterine body; this can be located by gentle pressure with the tip of the index finger.
- The plunger of the pipette should be firmly depressed to deposit the semen just into the uterine body.
- The pipette should be carefully withdrawn.
- Excessive palpation of the genital tract and ovaries should be discouraged.
- A dose of 20–30 × 10^6 spermatozoa is present in each straw, with between 6–7 × 10^6 alive after thawing.

Timing of insemination

Timing is important to ensure good pregnancy rates and is dependent upon accurate oestrus detection (see section 1.8). A cow first seen in oestrus in the morning should be inseminated that day (preferably in the afternoon), whilst if first seen in the afternoon or evening it should be inseminated the next morning. The optimum time is towards the end of oestrus or within several hours afterwards.

14.5 SELECTION AND CARE OF BULLS AT AI CENTRES

Bulls that are routinely used for semen collection at AI centres need to be in good physical condition, and to get plenty of exercise. Particular attention must be given to the state of the locomotor system, especially the feet. Firm but sympathetic handling and restraint are needed.

Bulls are examined by a veterinary officer of the Ministry of Agriculture, Fisheries and Food in order to reduce the possibility of the dissemination of undesirable genetic traits, and also because of the danger of the spread of venereally-transmitted and other diseases. Examination of the bull comprises an assessment of any anatomical defects that might be transmitted to its progeny and an evaluation of the herd of origin and any animals that may have been served by him. Tests for the presence of specific infectious agents such as *Mycobacterium tuberculosis, Brucella abortus Tritrichomonas fetus, Campylobacter fetus.* IBR, BVD and enzootic bovine leukosis are carried out, together with tests for other conditions that might affect the bull's health. Only when a veterinary certificate of freedom from infection is issued can a bull be moved to an authorised AI centre. There he remains in isolation for a further 60 days, during which time further tests are done, before he joins the bull stud.

Regular examinations for health are carried out by the veterinary officer responsible for the centre.

14.6 REGULATIONS CONCERNING THE USE OF AI IN THE UK

The Ministry of Agriculture, Fisheries and Food is responsible for the regulation of AI in the UK; readers are urged to consult the relevant acts and orders and should contact the appropriate veterinary officers for advice if required.

AI centres are approved by the Ministry of Agriculture, Fisheries and Food. A veterinary officer will visit the centres at three-monthly intervals to report on their organisation and conduct and on the technical efficiency of the inseminations. There is a statutory requirement to record details of the owner of the cow, and record cow and bull identity, at every insemination. All semen used in AI is deep-frozen and must be subjected to a 28-day quarantine period before use.

There are rigid controls on the importation of semen into the UK and many countries have strict requirements on the import of semen from the UK. Current regulations must be examined.

Do-it-yourself (DIY) AI is covered by separate regulations which allow farmers and their employees to perform AI on their own cattle with semen stored on the farm and subject to a licence issued by the Ministry of Agriculture, Fisheries and Food.

14.7 METHODS OF ASSESSING THE EFFICIENCY OF AI

Efficiency is measured by the 'non-return rate', which is the percentage of cows that have not returned to oestrus after a certain period of time since insemination – normally at intervals of 30–60 or 90–120 days.

The non-return rates are higher than the pregnancy rates (see section 7.10), which are a better measure, and should be between 70% and 80%. The discrepancy between pregnancy rates and non-return rates is due to:

- Failure to report return to oestrus before culling the cow.
- Use of natural service after failure of AI.
- Fetal death with return to oestrus outside normal time intervals (see section 8.1).
- Failure to detect returns to oestrus within normal time intervals.

14.8 POOR RESULTS FROM AI

These may be due to:

- Incorrect timing of AI (see sections 5.6 and 14.4).
- Incorrect or poor insemination technique, especially if DIY AI is used (see section 14.4).
- Poor storage and handling of semen, especially at thawing (see section 14.3).
- Vaginitis due to *Ureaplasma spp*. A narrow plastic sheath placed over the AI pipette can prevent uterine contamination.
- Variations in bull fertility.

15 Infertility in the Bull

15.1 GENERAL CONSIDERATIONS

When infertility is suspected in a herd in which natural service is used, the bull must always be suspected of being responsible. It is important to eliminate him as a cause before spending an inordinate amount of time investigating other likely causes; several examinations may be necessary before a specific diagnosis can be made (see sections 13.4–13.6);.

15.2 METHOD OF INVESTIGATION

A carefully planned and strict routine is necessary, as follows:

- Long-term history, namely age, breeding, source, duration of ownership and proof of fertility.
- Short-term history, for which good records are important, namely frequency of use, method of use, housing and feeding, handling, recent proof of fertility, and the precise observation and complaint about the bull.
- Detailed clinical examination of general health, especially of the genital system. The response of the bull to a cow or heifer in oestrus must be noted. His copulatory behaviour should, if possible, be closely observed and a semen sample must be collected and evaluated (see sections 13.4–13.7). Following this investigation it should be possible to categorise the reason for infertility into at least one of the following main causes: poor or no libido; impotence; reduced or no ability to fertilise; (these are described in sections 15.3–15.8).

15.3 LOSS OR LACK OF LIBIDO

Libido (sexual desire) varies greatly from breed to breed and within breeds. Generally beef bulls, which are phlegmatic, have poorer libido than dairy bulls.

The environment in which the bull is kept, the person handling the bull, the method used to restrain the bull and the place in which service takes place can have a profound influence on libido, although frequently a precise cause for poor libido cannot be determined. The following may be responsible:

- Age: libido declines in old bulls.
- Bullying: young bulls especially can be subjected to extensive bullying by groups of cows and heifers; this can have short-term and long-term effects upon libido.
- Noise and distractions.
- Unusual environments, handlers or methods of restraint.
- Boredom: some variation in service routine can be advantageous.
- Lack of exercise.
- Overweight.
- Severe debility.
- Over-use.
- Intercurrent disease.
- Severe pain to the locomotor system and back, and also to the penis where infectious agents such as BHV-1 (see section 8.7) can cause a severe inflammation and ulceration of the glans penis and prepuce (balanoposthitis).
- Rupture of corpus cavernosum penis (see sections 13.1 and 15.5).
- Uncertainty about foothold.
- Anabolic steroids.

Treatment of poor libido

In many cases this involves improved husbandry, sexual rest and treatment of intercurrent diseases. Bulls with inherently poor libido should not be used for breeding because of the possibility of the trait being inherited.

Treatment with gonadotrophins such as hCG or testosterone is of little value or may even be counterproductive.

15.4 IMPOTENCE

The bull has good libido but he does not serve the cow, i.e. he is impotent. An accurate and detailed description of the bull's behaviour at attempted service must be obtained. It may be necessary to observe the bull closely on several occasions.

15.5 IMPOTENCE ASSOCIATED WITH FAILURE TO PROTRUDE THE PENIS

- *Phimosis (stenosis of the preputial orifice).* On digital exploration the orifice should accept at least three fingers simultaneously. *Phimosis* may be congenital in young bulls and should not be treated surgically because it may be an inherited defect. It can be an acquired condition in young and other bulls because of over-use, trauma and chronic balanoposthitis.

- *Failure of erection.* This can be due to congenital or, less commonly, acquired vascular shunts, which allow blood to escape from the corpus cavernosum penis and thus prevent normal erection (see section 13.1). The partially protruded portion is limp and flaccid; there is no treatment. Occlusion of the longitudinal canals of the CCP can also be responsible.
- *Penile tumours,* usually fibropapillomas, which are quite common, can prevent protrusion if large.
- *Congenital shortening of the penis.* It is doubtful if this occurs or whether it is merely a failure of erection. The penis of the mature bull is about 90cm in length.
- *Adhesions between the penis and prepuce.* Chronic balanoposthitis due to trauma or infections such as BHV-1. Treatment by surgical separation of the adhesions is rarely successful.
- *Failure of separation of the penis and prepuce at puberty.*
- *Persistent frenulum.*
- *Rupture of the corpus cavernosum penis.* Usually diagnosed earlier because of the effect upon libido and evidence of pain. Swelling cranial to sigmoid flexure and scrotum.
- *Spiral deviation within the prepuce.* It can be intermittent within the prepuce, hence sometimes protrusion will occur. Movement of the erect penis can be seen and palpated within the prepuce.

15.6   IMPOTENCE ASSOCIATED WITH FAILURE OF INTROMISSION

The bull mounts and protrudes the penis but is incapable of intromission. This can be due to:

- *Spiral deviation of the penis (see section 15.5).* The penis normally spirals within the vagina after intromission; if it spirals before, then intromission is not possible. The penis is deflected ventrally and to the right and can become a complete anticlockwise spiral. It is due to slipping of the dorsal apical ligament of the penis. Surgical correction is possible, but should only be performed on bulls used for cross-breeding. It can occur intermittently.
- *Ventral deviation of the penis ('rainbow penis').* The penis is curved ventrally without spiralling; it is due to a weak dorsal apical ligament or occlusion of the longitudinal canals of CCP.
- *Persistent frenulum.* This can prevent complete protrusion or cause some degree of penile deviation. It is due to failure of complete separation of the penis and prepuce at puberty, and may be an inherited characteristic.
- *Large fibropapillomata.*

- *Indeterminable causes.* The penis appears to be normally erect and protruded, but intromission does not occur because of pain, poor foothold, disparity in the size of the cow or heifer, behavioural problems or neurological abnormalities.

15.7 IMPOTENCE ASSOCIATED WITH NON-EJACULATION

Intromission occurs but the bull does not thrust and ejaculate (see section 13.3).

It is usually impossible to determine the precise cause. It may be due to pain, poor foothold, a behavioural problem or neurological abnormalities resulting in a defective ejaculatory reflex. Treat with sexual rest and change the service routine.

15.8 REDUCTION IN, OR FAILURE OF, FERTILISATION

The bull has normal libido and is capable of normal copulation, but fertilisation fails to occur.

A detailed clinical examination of the genital system is necessary with semen collection and evaluation on at least three separate occasions at about 30-day intervals (see Chapter 13). Causes of poor semen quality are:

- *High environmental temperature.*
- *Intercurrent disease*, especially if there is pyrexia.
- *Stress* associated with transportation, a new environment or procedures such as casting and foot-trimming.
- *Over-use* (see section 13.8).
- *Infection of the genital system.* Pus may be seen in the ejaculate or large numbers of leucocytes in the semen smear. The site of infection may be the testes, epididymides or vesicular glands. Palpation will usually reveal pain or change in the consistency of the organ. Treatment is with prolonged antibiotic therapy.
- *Mastitis* of vestigial inguinal mammary glands.
- *Testicular hypoplasia.* This is observed in young bulls where the testes are small and soft, although the libido is normal; there is usually an aspermic ejaculate. It is possible that it is an inherited condition. There is no treatment.
- *Testicular degeneration.* There is a history of normal fertility followed by a gradual decline and ultimately complete failure to sire any calves. Libido is normal. Testes are small, initially soft, but then become shrunken and harder. Initially a poor ejaculate is obtained with low

sperm density and large numbers of dead and abnormal spermatozoa; eventually it is completely aspermic. There is no treatment.

- *Venereal diseases.* These are unlikely to have any effect upon the spermatozoa. Pregnancy fails to develop because of early embryonic death resulting from an unfavourable uterine environment (see sections 7.7, 7.9 and 8.2).
- *Segmental aplasia of Wolffian ducts.* Failure of embryological development of normal duct system which would enable transport of spermatozoa from testes. Unilateral aplasia would have little or no effect on fertility; bilateral would result in the bull being sterile from the age of puberty.
- *Morphologically abnormal spermatozoa.* Some defects occur because of rough or unsympathetic handling of the semen, others occur because of faults in spermatogenesis and sperm maturation. Interpretation of the significance of slight defects in sperm morphology requires the opinion of an expert.

Further reading

Arthur, G.H., Noakes, D.E., Pearson, H. and Parkinson, T.J. (1996) *Veterinary Reproduction and Obstetrics*, 7th edn. W.B. Saunders Co. London.

Cox, J.E. (1987) *Surgery of the Reproductive Tract in Large Animals*, 3rd edn. Liverpool University Press, Liverpool.

Esslemont, R.J. and Spincer, I. (1993) *Daisy Report No. 2*. University of Reading, Reading.

Esslemont, R.J. and Kossaibati, M.A. (1995) Daisy Report No. 4, University of Reading, Reading.

Lamming, G.E., Flint, A.P.F. and Weir, B.J. (eds) (1991) Reproduction in Domestic Ruminants II. *Journal of Reproduction and Fertility* (Suppl. 43).

Ministry of Agriculture, Fisheries and Food (1985) *Dairy Herd Fertility*. Book No. 259. Her Majesty's Stationery Office, London.

Niswender, G.D., Baird, D.T. and Findlay, J.K. (eds) (1987) Reproduction in Domestic Ruminants I. *Journal of Reproduction and Fertility* (Suppl. 34).

Peters, A.R. and Ball, P.J.H. (1995) *Reproduction in Cattle*, 2nd edn. Blackwell Science, Oxford.

Roberts, S.J. (1986) *Veterinary Obstetrics and Genital Diseases (Theriogenology)*, 3rd edn. Published by the author, Woodstock, Vermont.

Scaramuzzi, R.J., Nancarrow, C.D. and Doberska, C. (eds) (1995) Reproduction in Domestic Ruminants III. *Journal of Reproduction and Fertility* (Suppl. 49).

Index

Abortion
  causation 74–7
  definition 73
  frequency 73
  investigation 77–8
  legal requirements 74
Actinomyces pyogenes 75, 107–109
AI *see* artificial insemination
Allantochorion 29–31
  palpation 35, 36
Allantois 29, 30
Amnion 29, 30
Amorphous globosus 82
Ampullae 123, 126
Anasarca 95
Anoestrus 56
Anovulation 61
Arthrogryposis 79, 95
Artificial insemination 60, 129–34
  advantages 129
  disadvantages 129
  do-it-yourself 60, 133
  efficiency 134
  reasons for failure 134
  regulations 133
  technique 131–2
  timing 132
Ascites 95

Bacillus licheniformis 75
Balanoposthitis 136
Bovine Herpes Virus 1 72, 77
Bovine Viral Diarrhoea 72, 77
Breeding fitness of bull
  determination 125, 126
Brucella abortus 76
Brucellosis Orders

1979 (Scotland) 74
1981 (England and Wales) 74
Bühner's method 83, 84
Bulbo-urethral glands 122, 124

Caesarean section 91
Calf, new-born
  adaptation 44
  birth weight 37, 38
  examination 44, 45
  rejection by cow 45
  resuscitation 45
  weakly 45
Calving environment 41
Calving index 66
Calving interval 55, 65
Calving rate per insemination 54, 55
Calving-to-conception interval 66
Calving-to-first-service interval 67
Campylobacter fetus 72, 76
Cardiovascular defects 80
Caruncles 26, 36
  after calving 48, 49
  palpation 36
Cassou insemination pipette 131–2
'Casting calf bed' 105–7
CCP *see* corpus cavernosum penis
Cervix
  dilatation 40, 87
    incomplete 92, 97
  examination 15–17, 40
  involution 47
  palpation 17
  prolapse 82–4
Chlamydia psittaci, 72, 77
CIDR 13, 56
CL *see* corpus luteum

Cleft palate 79
Clenbuterol hydrochloride 43
Cloprostenol, dose rate 15
Conception rate *see* pregnancy rate
Congenital abnormalities 79–82, 94–5
Copulation 125
Corpus cavernosum penis 124
  rupture 136, 137
Corpus luteum
  after calving 47
  artificual shortening of lifespan 11,
      14, 15
  growth 4, 5, 6, 7, 8
  hormone production 7, 8
  in pregnancy 34
  palpation 20–22
  persistent 58
  ultrasonography 26, 27
Corticosteroids 39
  use in inducing lactation 52, 53
  use in inducing parturition 41, 42
Cotyledons 26, 30
  palpation 36
Crown-rump length 32
Culling
  due to fertility problems 54
  rate 68
Cumulus oophorus 5, 6
Cysts 22, 27, 57–8, 64, 66

Dinoprost, dose rate 15
Dioestrus 4
Disposition
  abnormal 95–7
    correction 88, 89
  normal 88, 89
Donor cows in embryo transfer
  preparation 112–13
  selection 111
Ductus deferens 122, 123
Dystocia
  definition 86
  incidence 86
  investigation 86–7

Ejaculation 125
  failure 138
Electro-ejaculation 126
Embryo
  collection 113–16

development 29, 32
  freezing 117
  micromanipulation 117
  recovery 116
  storage 117
  see also embryo transfer
Embryo transfer
  applications 110–111
  conduct of 111
  non surgical 116–17
  surgical 116
Embryonic death
  early 54–5, 63–4, 71–2
  late 54–5, 65, 71–2
Embryotomy 89
Endometritis, chronic 107–108
Endometrium 25
  regeneration 48–9
Epididymis 122–3
Episiotomy 103
Erection 124
  failure 137
'Estrumate' 15
Eye abnormalities 79

Fallopian tubes *see* uterine tubes
Fertility
  after calving 50
  definition 54
  evaluation in a herd 65–8
  expectations for 54–5
  maintenance 69–70
  monitoring 69–70
  records 69–70, 74
  see also infertility, pregnancy rate
Fertilization 28–9
  failure 54–5, 60–62, 138–9
Fetal fluids 31, 35
  excess production 85
Fetal membranes 29–31, 35
Fetal moles *see* Amorphous globosus
Feto-maternal disproportion 90–91
Fetotome 90
Fetotomy 89–91
Fetus
  death 55, 65, 72–78
  estimation of age 32
  growth 31–2
  maceration 78
  mummification 72–3

palpation 36
Fibropapilloma 137–8
Foley catheter 114–16
Follicle-stimulating hormone *see* FSH
Follicles 4–8
   after calving 46
   growth 4–5
   hormone production 7
   luteinized 20
   palpation 20
   ultrasonography 23, 26, 27
Freemartins 38, 56
Fremitus 36
Frenulum, persistent 137
FSH
   in ovarian function 6–8
   in spermatogenesis 121–22
   in superovulation 112–13
Fungi 76

Genital system, female 15–27
   contusions after calving 104
   external examination 15–16
   occlusion 60–61
   rectal palpation 17–23
   segmental aplasia 60
   ultrasonography of 23–7
   vaginal examination 16–17
Genital system, male 121–24
   clinical examination 125–6, 135
   infection 133, 138
Gestation length 37
Gluteal nerve paralysis 104
Graafian follicles *see* follicles

Haematomas 104
Haemophilus somnus 72, 77
'Hip lock' 92
Hormones *see under individual names*
Hydrocephalus 79
Hydrops allantois 85
Hydrops amnii 85

IBR, *see* bovine Herpes Virus 1
Impotence 136–8
Infertility, female
   definition 54
   investigation 55–68
Infertility, male 60, 135–9
   investigation 135

Inhibin 5, 122
Interferon 33
Interoestrous interval 4
   prolonged 65
   short 64
Intromission 125
   failure 137–8

KaMaR heat mount detectors 9, 10

Lactation
   artificial induction 52–3
   onset 51
Lactogenesis 51–2
Leptospira interrogans 75
Leydig cells 121–22, 123
LH
   in ovarian function 6–8
   in spermatogenesis 122
LHRH 6
Libido 124–5
   poor 135–6
Listeria monocytogenes 75
Luprostiol, dose rate 15
'Lutalyse' 15
Luteal deficiency 64
Luteinizing hormone *see* LH
Luteinizing-hormone-releasing
   hormone *see* LHRH
Luteolysis 7–8, 11

Maternal recognition of pregnancy 33
Mammary development 51
'Membrane slip' 35
Metoestrus 4
Metritis, acute 107
Milk let-down 52
Monsters 79–82, 94–5
Mounting response 9

Neosporum caninum 76–7
Nerve damage during calving 104
'Non-return rate' 134
'Norgestamet' 13–14
Nutrition
   relation to fertility 56, 63
Nymphomania 64

Obturator nerve paralysis 104
Oestradiol-17β 5, 7, 8

Oestradiol benzoate 12, 52, 53, 108
Oestradiol valerate 14
Oestriol 5
Oestrogens
    at parturition 39
    in mammary development 51
    in pregnancy 34
    see also individual hormones
Oestrone 5
    sulphate 36
Oestrous cycle
    artificial control 11–15
    hormonal changes 6–8
    stages 4
    see also ovarian activity, cyclical
Oestrus 4
    detection 8–11, 58
        efficiency 68–9
        rate 68
    duration 4, 8
    during pregnancy 34
    non-occurrence 55–9
    signs 8–9
    silent 9, 58
    synchronization 11–15
Oocytes 4, 5, 6
Organogenesis 29
Ovarian activity, cyclical 4
    hormonal control 5–8
    return after calving 46–7
    see also oestrous cycle
Ovarian bursa 18–19, 60–61
Ovaries
    agenesis 56
    changes during oestrous cycle 4–5
    hormones produced by 5–8
    hypoplasia 56
    palpation 18–23
    ultrasonography 26–7
Oviducts *see* uterine tubes
Ovulation 4–5
    after calving 46–7
    delayed 61–62
    rate 38, 110
    relation to oestrus 4, 7
Oxytocin 6, 7–8, 39, 52

Palpation, rectal 17–23
    to diagnose pregnancy 34–6
    to investigate infertility 55–6

Parturition
    delaying 43
    first stage 40, 88
    induction 41–3
    initiation 39
    second stage 40, 88
    signs 39
    third stage 40–41, 99
Pelvis
    bony defects 93
    examination 16
Penis 124, 126
    adhesions 137
    congenital shortening 137
    failure to protrude 136–7
    spiral deviation 137
    tumours 137, 138
    ventral deviation 137
Perineum
    examination 16
    lacerations 102–3
Perosomus elumbus 95
$PGF_2\alpha$ *see* prostaglandin $F_2\alpha$
Phimosis 136–7
Placenta 32–3, 40
    expulsion 40, 99–100
    retention 99–101
'Planipart' 43
Pneumovagina 17, 62, 103
Polydactyly 79
Polyspermy 29
Position
    abnormal 96
    dorsal 88
Posture
    abnormal 95–6
    extended 88
Pregnancy
    diagnosis 33–6
    duration 37
    endocrinology 33
Pregnancy rate 67–8
    after artificial insemination 134
    after calving 50
    after synchronization of oestrus 15
Pregnancy-specific protein B 35
PRID 12
Presentation
    abnormal 96–7
    anterior longitudinal 88

Progestagens 11–14
Progesterone 4, 5, 6–8
    at parturition 39, 51
    in mammary development 51
    in pregnancy 33, 34
    milk concentration assay 34–5
    use in synchronizing oestrus 12–13
Progesterone-releasing intravaginal
        device *see* PRID
Prolactin 7, 34, 51
Prolapse
    cervico-vaginal 82–3, 84
    uterine 105–7
Pro-oestrus 4
'Prosolvin' 15
Prostaglandin F$_2\alpha$ 7, 39, 47–8
    use in inducing parturition 41–3
    use in synchronizing oestrus 11,
        14–15
Prostate gland 122, 123
Puberty
    female 3, 55
        delayed 56
    male 124–5
Puerperium, definition 46
Pyometra 58–9, 108–9

Recipient cows in embryo transfer
    preparation 113
    selection 111
Retained foetal membranes *see*
        placenta retention
Rolling 94

Salmonella spp. 75
Schistosoma reflexus 79, 80, 95
Scoliosis 79, 95
Semen
    collection 126–7, 130
    composition 127
    evaluation 128
    freezing 130–131
    importation 133
    poor quality 138–9
    processing 130–131
    thawing 131
Seminal vesicles 123–4
Seminiferous tubules 121, 123
Service, natural
    frequency 128

Speculum, vaginal 16–17
Spermatogenesis 121, 123
Spermatozoa 121, 122, 123
    abnormal 128, 139
    capacitation 21–2
    concentration 127, 128
    evaluation 128
    motility 128
    output 127
Sterility, definition 54
Stillbirth 78
Subfertility 54
Submission rate 68
Super-ovulation 112–13
Synchronisation of oestrus 11–15
Syndactyly 79

Tail paint 9
Teaser cows 126, 130
Testes 121, 128
    degeneration 138
    hypoplasia 138
Testosterone 122
Torticollis 79, 95
Traction 89
Traction ratio, calculation 91–2
Triplets, incidence 38, 110
Tritrichomonas fetus 72, 76
Tunica albuginea 121, 124
Twinning
    incidence 38, 110
    induced 110, 117
Twins
    conjoined 79, 80, 95
    simultaneous presentation 94

Ultrasonography 23–7
Urovagina 62
Uterine horns 18
    during pregnancy 35–6
    palpation 18
Uterine tubes 4, 18, 19
    palpation 18
Uterus
    bacterial contamination after
        parturition 49–50
    inertia 97–8
    infection 58, 62, 63–4, 69, 107–9
    involution 47–8
    prolapse 105–7

rupture 84, 97
tears 104–5
tone 18
torsion 83, 93–4, 97
ventral deviation 98

Vagina
artificial 126–7, 130
discharge 21, 49, 107
examination 16–17, 107–8
lacerations 102–3
palpation 17
prolapse 82–3, 84

stricture 93
Vesicular glands 122, 123–4
Vulva
discharge 107
examination 16
lacerations 102–3
stricture 93

'Waterbag' 40
Wolffian ducts
segmental aplasia 139

Zona pellucida 6, 29